Leaky Gut Syndrome

The Invisible Thief
That Steals Your Health and
Wellbeing
and
What to do about it!

Charlotte Alexander

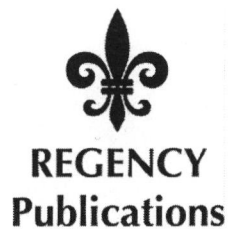

REGENCY
Publications

Leaky Gut Syndrome

ISBN-13: 978-0615800479 (Regency Publications)

ISBN-10: 0615800475

Contents

"He, who has health, has hope; and he who has hope,
has everything."

Thomas Carlyle

Introduction:
The Thief Within

What if I told you there is an invisible thief that can enter your life and steal your wellbeing? This thief is a chameleon—with many identities—but always insidious and greedy. He is Leaky Gut. His loot? Your good health.

I was robbed by this devious thief and suffered with leaky gut syndrome for more than 20 years. I had no idea what was happening to me as I endured the nagging, chronic symptoms that seemed to take over my life.

My symptoms were many including: abdominal pain, irritable bowel syndrome, extreme allergies (I was diagnosed with 49 different ones), food intolerances, migraines, Candida, and dermatitis so severe that I had to wear two pairs of gloves to do the dishes—rubber gloves to protect me from the dishwater, and white cotton gloves inside the rubber gloves to protect me from the latex.

My unrelated symptoms were indeed a puzzle for allopathic (conventional) doctors. One told me it was all in my head, others prescribed medications that simply didn't work. Each tried to treat different symptoms, but never the underlying cause. I was misdiagnosed for many years.

What about you?

Has the same thing happened to you, too? Have you been suffering for far too long—visiting too many specialists—and spending a great deal of time and money? Have you felt like throwing your hands up in disgust and saying there's no hope of ever feeling better?

Don't give up! You and I both know that the failure of many conventional doctors to recognize and diagnose this disorder doesn't make it any less real.

There's help for you

It took me a long time to find a medical doctor to help me. I found a physician who specializes in integrated medicine (a healing-oriented medical approach that takes into account the whole of a person—the body, mind and spirit).

This doctor was the first to tell me about leaky gut syndrome and its effects. With his diagnosis, suddenly all my diverse symptoms made sense. The long-term result of a leaky gut is the development of autoimmune diseases, which means the body is attacking its own tissues. I indeed was suffering from various autoimmune diseases.

Your leaky gut

If you have leaky gut syndrome, you know the major toll it takes on your health and wellbeing. You know the limitations it puts on your body. Your symptoms may not be the same as mine; there are more than eighty recognized autoimmune diseases, including some as common as allergies, or as painful and stubborn as fibromyalgia. But whatever your chronic health issues and symptoms are, you know they're affecting your quality of life.

What if you could experience health, vitality and energy again?

That's what this book is all about. It's your personal resource and reference manual to help you understand the complexity of leaky gut syndrome. It's also chockfull of advice (that you can start using immediately) to help you identify and overcome this complex health concern.

I bet at some point, you too have probably been told that there is nothing basically wrong with you. If you've been on the same journey as I have, and haven't been able to find a solution, this book is indeed for you. I don't want anyone else to ever go through what I've been through—the twenty plus years of searching for help to feel better.

I've not only detailed what leaky gut is and what causes it, but I've even devoted a chapter to how your personal healthcare provider goes about making a definitive, accurate diagnosis.

You can have the quality of life you deserve. You just need the straight facts. You're going to get them **here!**

Diagnosis: The first step in healing

Once you have a diagnosis in hand, then leaky gut becomes far less mysterious and menacing. An accurate diagnosis also means the beginning of an effective treatment plan. Because, once you know you're suffering from leaky gut, you can take the necessary steps to overcome it.

And yes, I've provided you with a *variety* of ways that you can start healing your body. From diet to dietary supplements to herbs and beyond, you can choose the solutions that work for your specific, individual health problems.

Visit your healthcare provider before you begin

I have one word of caution. Before you embark on any program, you need to consult a healthcare provider. Look for medical doctors specializing in integrated medicine, as I did, or naturopathic physicians or other alternative health professionals to help guide you.

Make your best effort to find the right resources and the best fit for you. Finding the specific guidance you need is key. Your determination will be worth it. It's time to quit suffering and find something I suspect you haven't experienced in a long time…Hope.

Chapter 1
What Is Leaky Gut Syndrome?

L eaky what? If you've never heard the term before, you might be thinking it's a ridiculous name for a medical condition. Leaky gut syndrome (LGS) is also known as the more conventional-sounding "increased intestinal permeability."

But regardless of the name used to describe the condition, the fact is the allopathic (conventional) medical community, for the most part, refuses to acknowledge this far-too-common condition.

You'll need to look to medical doctors who specialize in integrated medicine, naturopathic physicians, or other natural healthcare practitioners who are experienced in treating leaky gut for help.

Picturing leaky gut

I'm going to describe leaky gut syndrome in detail. But before I do, it might be helpful to have a visual to make it easier to understand.

Imagine the lining of your small intestine like a window screen that lets air in and keeps bugs out. When leaky gut comes along, it punches holes in the screen.

Ever sit out on a screened porch at night? If mosquitoes can find a way through the screen, those nasty things will bite you. It's the same for your body. When the lining of your intestine becomes irritated and inflamed, the mucous lining of your small intestine becomes too porous (leaky).

Bacteria, other toxins, microorganisms, food particles and pathogens get into your blood stream, wreaking havoc. The presence of these toxins triggers an autoimmune reaction in which the immune system attacks your own cells. And this can eventually cause a host of gastrointestinal problems, not the least of which are abdominal bloating, excess gas and cramps.

But there are other ways this situation can affect your body as well, including causing fatigue, food sensitivities, and joint pain. Many of these so-called symptoms show up as a variety of conditions we consider disorders and diseases in and of themselves. Linking them to leaky gut syndrome is not usually what people think of doing. Listed below are just a handful of these symptoms:

Symptoms of leaky gut

- Alcohol use

- Autoimmune diseases

- Candida

- Certain medications

- Chronic constipation

- Chronic stress

- Environmental toxins

- Excessive consumption of processed foods

- Food sensitivities

- Low-fiber diet

- Low stomach acid

- Nutritional deficiencies

- Severe burns

Many times we treat these symptoms as disorders. We treat them, but don't realize why they exist to begin with. The truth of the matter is that, as the toxins in your blood take hold, they eventually affect other parts of your body, many of which are still banding together trying hard to keep you healthy.

Leaky gut syndrome and your liver

Among the first of your organs affected is your liver. The more toxins that enter your system, the more your liver works at excreting them. Yes, this does keep the organ active—very active. If left untreated, the liver gets overloaded and can no longer detoxify these materials. As a result, they're returned to the blood to circulate.

One of the tasks your blood performs is maintenance of something the medical community calls "chemical homeostasis." Through this mechanism, your body attempts to maintain an internal stability. It deftly coordinates the responses of various actions of different organs throughout your system. If, for any reason, the balance is disturbed, the poisonous chemicals and some physical debris get delivered to into what's called the tissue matrix.

Giving its all: the lymph system

And that's where another organ jumps into action, trying to maintain a healthy balance. It's your lymph system, a vital part of your immune system.

Even though your lymphatic system tries to collect and then neutralize these toxins, it isn't always successful. The burden is then placed on the liver and the tissue matrix, which have the potential to turn toxic.

It takes some time, but eventually what initially was merely a "gut-barrier" issue has escalated into tissue toxicity. And this, in turn, can trigger a chain reaction of other problems. If your tissue environment is compromised, bacteria grow.

Not only that, but the lymph fluids in your body accumulate causing lymphatic swelling. You'll soon recognize this by the presence of inflammation in your body. This swelling is what causes the multitude of possible symptoms, some of which go unexplained.

The consequences of toxin buildup

Let's take this situation one step further. If too many toxins accumulate, the immune system exhausts itself working against them. This means that, in all likelihood, a portion of the toxins inevitably enter the body. At the same time, the process also depletes your immune system.

You may wonder why the immune system is affected. It's a little known fact (and now one you're in on) that seventy percent of your immune system is actually located in and around your digestive system.

This portion of the system is called "gut-associated lymphatic tissues," or "GALT." These tissues are located in the lining of the digestive tract and in the intestinal mucus.

What happens when the liver is overwhelmed?

This condition can literally overwhelm your liver, leaving it unable to process everything efficiently. When this happens, the liver then turns to your immune system for help. Unfortunately, we've already established that your immune response is stressed, and unable to act as it should.

The bacteria then accumulate to unhealthy levels, and this opens the door for opportunistic infections to appear. These are infections you normally wouldn't develop. Due to the severely weakened state of your immune system, they "sneak in."

Another organ then becomes affected by this overrun of bacteria. Your adrenal glands, two small glands sitting atop each of your kidneys, are vital in resisting infection. The prolonged presence of leaky gut syndrome eventually

— and slowly — reduces the healthy function of these glands as well.

In the initial stages, there is no adrenal excess. This can be easily tested by measuring your cortisol output—the hormone the adrenal glands produce. But, as the syndrome continues unabated, cortisol levels increase. And that's when a condition called "adrenal exhaustion" occurs.

Briefly, just a few of the symptoms indicating you may be experiencing adrenal fatigue include: exhaustion, sleep that doesn't refresh you, inability to cope with stress, difficulty concentrating and poor digestion.

How leaky gut syndrome reveals itself

Now that you understand — at least in general terms — how this syndrome develops, hopefully you have a greater appreciation for how all the parts of your body work together to help fight off disease. In the same way, your system teams up to create health. It's a two-way street.

It may not come as a surprise to you to discover that leaky gut syndrome can manifest itself in any number of ways in your system. While you can't call these "symptoms," they are indeed real health conditions. But the underlying cause of these conditions may very well be the presence of leaky gut syndrome.

In the next chapter, I discuss some of the factors that can cause leaky gut syndrome. Knowing what triggers this syndrome can help you take action to remedy it.

Chapter 2
The Causes of Leaky Gut Syndrome No One Talks About

By this time, you may have already approached a natural health practitioner or a naturopathic doctor who suspects that you may indeed have leaky gut syndrome. Probably your immediate question was, "What caused it?"

If only there were a simple one- or two-word answer to that question, but there isn't. In fact, there are a host of possible causes of this syndrome. And there are "hidden" causes that many don't even seem to talk about.

Therefore, if you're waiting for your healthcare provider to hand over one cause on a silver platter — well, unfortunately, that's not going to happen. More often than not, discovering the cause is sometimes the most difficult part of treating the syndrome.

Of course, you know your body better than anyone else. You know your health habits. And armed with this intimate information, when you're presented with a list of possible hidden causes, you may be able to identify the most likely causes for your body and check them out.

Common Causes of leaky gut syndrome

Here are just a few of the more common causes of this syndrome:

- Chronic use of NSAIDs

- Dysbiosis

- Candida

- Cancer therapy

- Chronic stress

- Environmental toxins

- Diet

- Aging

- Endotoxins

- AIDS

- Gastrointestinal disease

- Immune system overload

- Lack of Secretory IgA

- Abuse of alcohol

- Trauma

- Chronic infections

NSAIDs as a cause

NSAIDs (nonsteroidal anti-inflammatory drugs, (pronounced en-saids), are   medications used primarily to treat inflammation, mild to moderate pain, and fever.

They include such drugs as aspirin, Celebrex, ibuprofen, naproxen, Toradol, Lodine, Indocin, and more.

The success of NSAIDs lies in their ability to block tiny messengers known as *prostaglandins.* These substances circulate throughout your body and block pain and inflammation. But the work of these drugs doesn't end there.

The prostaglandins have another job. They're charged with healing and repairing your body. When you take an NSAID, you indeed are blocking the pain and giving yourself much-needed relief. But you're also effectively blocking any healing or repair process that needs to be performed.

That's right. Regardless of their tasks, though, the over-the-counter medication indiscriminately blocks all of the transmitters.

The digestive tract repairs itself every three days

The digestive tract repairs and replaces itself every three to five days. So you can see how the extended use of NSAIDs blocks the needed repair process. Eventually, the lining of the tract weakens, becomes inflamed, and then leaks. And the result — you have leaky gut syndrome.

Not only that, but prolonged use of NSAIDs raises your risk of developing ulcers of the stomach and the duodenum.

Want more reasons to reduce your dependency on them? This class of medication causes bleeding, damage to the mucus membranes of your intestines and gastrointestinal inflammation.

Additionally, NSAID use can lead to colitis and relapses of ulcerative colitis. Who knew that these easily accessible, almost ubiquitous pills everyone takes with barely a second thought could be so potentially troublesome?

Dysbiosis

If you're like me, you've probably never heard of the term "dysbiosis." The word was created by Dr. Eli Metchnikoff, a 1908 Nobel Prize winner, for his work on friendly bacterial flora.

You're already aware of the need to keep a balance between the harmful or pathogenic bacteria — as they're called in the medical community — and the helpful bacteria, often called *flora*.

When this balance is disrupted and your body contains more harmful than friendly bacteria, this state is called dysbiosis. It's derived from the word *symbiosis*, which means "living in harmony" and the prefix *dys* which means "not."

Dr. Metchnikoff discovered the natural bacteria of yogurt can prevent and actually reverse bacterial infections. Not only that, but thanks to his research, he revealed that the bacteria in yogurt has the ability to displace quite a few organisms which produce disease. Additionally, the yogurt bacteria content could also reduce the amount of accompanying toxins.

Given the state of modern medicine at the turn of the 20th century, this represented an amazing advance in the treatment of bacterial infections.

With the advent of antibiotics and immunizations, though, his research seemed far less important and…well, quite frankly, outdated. Until recently, that is.

A host of new laboratory testing and corresponding research created a revival in the interest of the topic.

Menacing microbes and your health

Medical science is discovering microbes that don't belong in the digestive tract. And why is this of interest? The microbes very often form chemicals toxic to the cells which are located around them. But that's only part of the increase in interest. These microbes can also be a source of poison to you.

The overrun of microbes places the lining of your intestines at risk. The probable consequence? The creation of a vast array of potentially dangerous substances, including secondary bile acids, amines, phenols ammonia, indoles, and hydrogen sulfide.

In turn, these substances may damage your intestinal lining by injuring the brush borders. The brush borders are the largest manufacturer of digestive enzymes in your small intestine. Eventually the damaged brush borders enzymes may be absorbed into your bloodstream.

Unfortunately, the adverse toll they're taking on your body isn't recognized immediately. After a while they can cause chronic conditions, many of which never get diagnosed.

So what's the ultimate cause of dysbiosis? We've already talked about it: the overuse of medications. But the extended use of NSAIDs is only one trigger to the development of the buildup of bad bacteria. We'll discuss the other class of drugs which can trigger this state next.

Those antibiotics that get me well?

Surely you must be mistaken. Antibiotics help to improve my health. They cure my infections — all sorts of infections. I get them when I have swollen glands. Well, you get the idea. They're a modern-day marvel.

Yes, I agree and there's where the problem comes in. The medical community has been depending on this simply amazing type of medication for just about every ailment you can imagine. Most patients practically demand some sort of antibiotics when they walk into a doctor's office complaining of an ailment, even if they don't suffer from a bacterial infection. Doctors, for their part, readily agree.

When good antibiotics go bad

But consider this. When you put antibiotics in your body, you're potentially disturbing the balance of intestinal microbes. Antibiotics, just like NSAIDs, really don't discriminate in their attack of bacteria. They kill the bad bacteria — the ones causing your ailment — as well as your friendly flora.

As a result, your system may be exposed to resistant bacteria (those that antibiotics can't seem to kill effectively), fungi, parasites, and viruses. Normally, a healthy balanced gut can keep this array of intruders at bay, thanks to the presence of friendly flora.

When the balance tilts toward the more harmful bacteria, the results can be irritation, inflammation and, given enough time, the presence of disease.

The most common microbe to appear because of this imbalance is the yeast infection *Candida,* a fungus.

You mean my Candida can be caused by leaky gut syndrome?

Yes, if you've ever suffered from a Candida infection then you know first-hand what the state of dysbiosis feels like—at least one type of imbalance.

Candida is a fungus that just about everyone carries around with them. But usually your system only contains small amounts, not enough to spark an infection. This small quantity is easily kept under control thanks to your friendly flora in conjunction with a strong immune system and a balanced intestinal pH.

The firm grasp of Candida

If this delicate balance is disturbed, the Candida takes advantage by growing and overrunning certain areas of your digestive tract. But their presence goes quite a bit deeper than that. These fungi create a chemical—acid protease—which "steals" the secretory IgA from the mucus membranes.

Secretory IgA is the secreted form of an antibody in the blood called IgA. IgA is produced in the blood, taken into the gut and secreted across the mucosal lining into that mucous layer that is the surface lining of our digestive tract. It's the mucosal immune barrier or first-line immune defense.

If the secretory IgA is depleted, it allows the Candida to anchor into and eventually continue to accumulate on your mucus membrane. Now the infection is firmly entrenched.

If that wasn't bad enough, once anchored and firmly in place, the Candida leaks toxins that leak into the bloodstream. Once circulating throughout your body, the toxins not only depress your immune system, but they also play havoc with the hormonal balance of your system and even disturb the healthy functioning of your brain.

What's next? How about increased food sensitivity?

Once Candida passes through your intestinal lining, antibodies then naturally respond by alerting your immune system to the presence of certain foods, which in turn increases your sensitivity to these foods. Later in this chapter we'll discuss the difference between food sensitivity and a true food allergy. (Yes, there's a difference.)

Most people acquire this infection through the prolonged use of antibiotics and steroid medications.

Many women develop it through the continued use of birth control pills. And still others find that the consumption of alcohol can trigger this condition.

How to tell if you have a Candida infection

So, how can you recognize a Candida infection? Could you be walking around with one right now without even knowing it? It's possible. Some of the more obvious symptoms include:

- Abdominal bloating

- Anxiety

- Constipation or Diarrhea (or both)

- Depression

- Sensitivities to the environment

- Fatigue

- Food sensitivities

- Foggy thought processes

- Insomnia

- Low blood sugar

- Mood swings

- Premenstrual syndrome

- Chronic vaginal infections

- Recurrent bladder infections

• Tinnitus

Granted, any one of these symptoms can indicate other underlying health problems, as well as the presence of a yeast infection. And that's exactly why Candida can be difficult to diagnose — and goes unnoticed for so long.

Steroid drugs and leaky gut syndrome

Most people, at some time or another, have used steroids. They're effective on many stubborn lingering health conditions and chronic health problems. They're most effective on allergies, inflammation, and autoimmune diseases. Prolonged use of steroids, though, eventually weakens your immune system. And yes, you already know this can cause trouble.

Your depressed immune system allows for the development of a fungal infection, not only in your gastrointestinal tract, but in just about every other part of your body as well.

Talk about side effects

It's like kicking a person when he's already down. You're dealing with strong cancer therapy drugs through chemotherapy. Or you may be undergoing radiation treatment. Perhaps both.

The last thing you need is to be told that these same drugs may be igniting the development of leaky gut syndrome. Unfortunately, it's true. Each of these treatments holds the possibility of disturbing the balance of your gastrointestinal tract. And that means you may eventually acquire a problem with absorbing foods.

This isn't just speculation. The disruption of this finely tuned balance is actually well documented in medical literature.

Got stress? Think leaky gut syndrome

It's true, chronic stress affects your immune system — and not for the better. It depresses your ability to fight off infections as well as retarding the healing process of wounds and injuries. When under stress, your body reduces its production of secretory IgA and DHEA, an adrenal hormone that delays the aging process and helps you handle stress.

Excessive stress also slows the digestive process, reduces blood flow to your digestive organs and eventually contributes to the manufacturing of toxic metabolites. Metabolites are substances crucial to your metabolism.

Since stress is so much a part of our lives, I've dedicated an entire chapter to various methods that can help you intelligently manage the stress in your life. This chapter alone may be invaluable to helping you improve your leaky gut syndrome.

When the environment attacks you

Believe it or not, it occurs on a daily basis. And not just to other people. You, too, are affected daily... hour by hour... even minute by minute... by the environment. Oh, I'm not talking about safely soaking up the warming rays of the sun and feeling great. I'm talking about some serious adverse effects that could be harming your body even as you read this.

Some natural health practitioners and environmentalists say you could be exposed to hundreds of household irritants, dangerous chemicals, environmental chemicals and toxic metals every day.

Even though you may not realize it, this near constant barrage is overloading your immune system. It also prevents your system from repairing itself from this exposure.

One of the first consequences of this situation is the breaking down of your connective tissue. Soon after that, your body begins lacking in various trace minerals like calcium, potassium, and magnesium.

This, in turn, causes acidosis within your cells and the swelling of tissues and cells.

Your diet as a source of leaky gut syndrome

Now, we're getting somewhere. It's time to look at one cause of leaky gut syndrome over which you have control. Your diet. I won't delve deeply into this topic here, because I've devoted an entire chapter to rebalancing your system through changes in your eating habits.

One of the problems with the American diet is its distinct lack of fiber. When you eat a diet that is deficient in fiber, you are effectively promoting a prolonged transit time — a situation that's not conducive to proper digestion.

Not only does this slowing of delivery hinder your bowel movements, but it also practically invites toxic byproducts to accumulate and irritate your gut.

Among the worst culprits are processed foods. These foods are usually filled with artificial additives, many of which are toxic according to resent medical research.

Be sure to check out the chapter on rebalancing your system through your diet. It'll help work wonders in healing your leaky gut syndrome.

The difference between food sensitivity and allergy

The exact link between food sensitivities and leaky gut syndrome can be a conundrum. It's difficult even for the best nutritionists to decide which health problem cropped up first.

Did your leaky gut syndrome cause your food sensitivities? Or did your food sensitivities trigger the leaky gut syndrome? One thing is fairly certain: the two seem to go hand-in-hand.

Many individuals confuse food sensitivity with a true food allergy. The two are not the same.

Let's start with food allergies, as you're probably more acquainted with them. One of the most common of these — especially among children — is the allergy to peanuts. Think about it. An allergy to peanuts evokes an immediate response in the body.

The first difference then is the reaction time. Food allergies, also known as "type 1 or immediate hypersensitivity reaction," trigger the response of a certain specific type IgE antibody. This antibody bonds to the food antigens which then release substances called cytokines. And this results in a number of true allergic symptoms: hives; itching, runny nose; and perhaps a skin rash.

Some individuals experience more serious consequences: respiratory distress, the closing of the throat, asthma, and even anaphylactic shock. A life-threatening condition, anaphylactic shock — or anaphylaxis — is an extremely serious reaction that affects your entire body. After being exposed to peanuts, let's say, your immune system becomes sensitized to it. Another exposure to it may illicit this dangerous allergic reaction.

The most critical aspect of food allergies is the extremely fast response your body has. Many times it happens within minutes, which means you must not only be aware of the contact with the allergen immediately, but be ready to act quickly.

Your physician can diagnose food allergies through patch skin tests and specific blood testing.

So do I have food sensitivity?

It's very possible. The first hallmark of food sensitivity is that very often the effects of it are not immediately apparent. This shows up in its medical name "delayed hypersensitivity reaction."

From the moment you eat the food to the time your reactions surface may take anywhere from two to three hours, or two to three days. As you may suspect, detecting this cause and effect is sometimes difficult.

Not only that, but the symptoms run the gamut, which makes the sensitivity hard to recognize.

Sensitivity occurs when the food particles escape through the damaged mucosal membranes, entering directly into the blood stream.

Your body views these food particles as foreign substances, which signals your immune system to spring into action. At the same time, the liver reacts. It too believes these antigens are toxic. The liver initiates the process of breaking them down.

When you continue to eat these foods, you only increase the permeability of your intestines. A vicious circle then develops, because you'll surely acquire even more food sensitivities over time.

Individuals are sensitive to any number of foods, but the following sources account for nearly eighty percent of the adverse reactions: beef, citrus fruits, dairy products, eggs, pork, and wheat.

Perhaps you suspect your health condition — or multiple conditions — are caused ultimately by your leaky intestinal lining. Your next move is to visit a physician who believes that this syndrome actually exists.

He or she can run you through a battery of diagnostic tests to accurately determine your status.

What kind of tests? Follow me to the next chapter.

Chapter 3
Diagnosing Leaky Gut Syndrome

Beginning to think leaky gut syndrome lies at the bottom of your varied health problems? Are some of these symptoms and conditions — from Candida yeast infections to food sensitivities — sounding familiar?

To be completely certain, you should consider getting a thorough diagnosis. That's all well and good. But just where do you begin?

Start by approaching a healthcare practitioner you trust and who understands the development of leaky gut syndrome.

Lactulose-mannitol test

The first step in diagnosing the condition is undergoing a lactulose-mannitol test. You may also hear this test referred to as the "PolyetheGlycol Test" or "PEG." Water-soluble sugar molecules, both mannitol and lactulose, can't be used or metabolized by your body. They differ in size and weight and are absorbed into your bloodstream. The actual rate of absorption varies.

In a healthy digestive process, the cells digest mannitol with ease. On the other hand, the lactulose only digests partially. Therefore, the results of this test should indicate a high level of mannitol and a low level of lactulose for a digestive system that isn't hindered by leaky gut syndrome.

If the opposite is true — low mannitol and high lactulose — it indicates the presence of leaky gut syndrome.

There's also a third possibility. Your test reveals low levels of both of the sugar molecules. This means you probably have a problem dealing with absorption.

Interestingly, many individuals with a high lactulose level and low mannitol — most likely leaky gut syndrome — also suffer with Celiac disease (the inability to digest gluten in wheat and other products), Crohn's disease, and ulcerative colitis.

The home test kit

If you prefer not to visit a doctor to undergo this test, a home kit is available. You simply follow the instructions and send it off to a pre-designated lab for analysis.

The test isn't difficult or complicated to do. You'll first collect a urine sample. This provides the lab with a baseline reading. You'll then drink a mannitol-lactulose solution. After waiting for six hours, you'll collect a second urine sample. You send these to the lab designated in your instructions. The results will reveal your levels. You'll also receive information on reading the results properly.

If the test indicates the development of leaky gut syndrome, you'll want to undergo several more tests, some of which look for a few other health conditions as well.

Is dysbiosis present?

One of these tests is called a "comprehensive digestive stool analysis." This test, many times abbreviated CDSA, reveals the bacterial balance (or imbalance) of your digestive tract. In effect, it detects if dysbiosis is present. That is the technical term for the imbalance. Not only that, but the test reviews the overall state of your digestive health.

It also performs a useful third function. It determines the presence — and possible level — of Candida in your system. If you recall the presence of this fungal infection is closely linked to leaky gut syndrome.

If this yeast infection is present, your healthcare provider will take a culture to determine the amount of growth and to determine a method for treating it.

But the CDSA is also a valuable tool in even more ways. It also measures the status of several digestive functions, including the digestion of proteins, fats, and carbohydrates. This valuable test also measures your level of a pancreatic enzyme called "cholecystokinin" and the quantity of short-chain fatty acids, as well as the level of butyric acid in your colon.

Despite these seemingly unpronounceable names, the issue really isn't all that complicated.

According to MayoClinc.com, cholecystokinin is a substance that enables the gallbladder to contract. It also triggers the pancreas to produce enzymes, both of which are essential for proper digestion. Butyric acid helps with raising your metabolism, controlling inflammation and helping you manage your stress.

Testing for what? Parasites?

Parasites don't sound very pleasing, but it's a fact: approximately one in six individuals carries at least one parasite according to the Centers for Disease Control. This is probably the highest this figure has ever been.

The presence of parasites has increased dramatically for several reasons. Contaminated water supplies, the increase and ease of international travel, the growth in day care centers with dozens of children being in contact with each other and sharing toys, and living closer to our pets are just a few of the many possible reasons for the burgeoning parasite population.

For the most part, you may never realize you have a parasite living off of you. But if you listen closely to your body, it's giving you subtle clues. So subtle, in fact, that they can all too easily be ignored or even mistaken for signals of other health issues.

Just a glance at the list below and you'll see exactly what I mean. These are a few of the indicators of the presence of these tiny creatures.

• Stomach pain

- Muscle aches

- Anemia

- Joint pain

- Bloating

- Itching

- Bloody stool

- Gas

- Coughing

- Unexplained weight loss

- Nervousness

- Unexplained fevers

- Pain

- Teeth Grinding

- Weakened Immune system

- Sleep problems

- Rashes

You can see the symptoms are wide ranging, to say the least. Not only that, but they could be attributed to any number of other more common health issues. That's exactly why the presence of parasites is so difficult to detect. Very often, parasites aren't even considered as a cause of any of these symptoms.

Random stool samples?

Some natural health physicians test for parasites — also called "parasitology tests" — using random stool samples. This method is far from perfect, though. In some instances, it's not very accurate; sometimes the test needs to be performed several times before any definitive diagnosis can be made.

Many parasites aren't lingering in your lower intestines and won't show up in a random stool sample. Many are instead located farther up along your digestive tract. In these cases, stool testing would reveal a negative result.

Physicians then give you an oral laxative inducing diarrhea, which pushes the parasite along the tract and out, so it does show up in your stool if it's present. Some physicians completely bypass the stool sample and instead use a rectal swab.

Of course, to get the most accurate diagnosis, go to a lab specializing in parasitology testing.

Anything else I should get tested?

Yes, we're not quite done yet. There are several more tests to ensure a completely accurate diagnosis, at least if you believe you have any sensitivities to food or chemicals. As you know, these are two indications that you may be suffering from leaky gut syndrome.

Many natural health professionals can provide you with testing in this realm. Identifying the specific foods or chemicals aggravating your system can greatly improve your chances of healing your health condition.

In fact, there are two methods of testing for these: an elimination diet and a provocation diet. I'll talk more about healing through these methods in a later chapter.

Another test for food sensitivities

In addition to the two diets, there are also a few blood tests which can be easily performed to help uncover sensitivities. These work by measuring your body's reaction to antibodies. These same tests are also useful for food allergies and sensitivities to environmental issues.

But you'll need to find a lab that tests specifically for IgG or IgG4 antibodies. Some labs also include testing for IgA, IgE, and IgM.

These are all tests that need to be conducted by your physician. He or she will be able to interpret the results. Included in this analysis, some labs even forward you a list of recommendations, including a suggestion to avoid the most troublesome prepared foods. You may also receive a rotation diet plan and other literature on the subject.

One last test

It's about time, you're thinking. But I did say that detecting leaky gut syndrome wasn't a simple, cut-and-dried diagnosis.

Your doctor may suggest one final test. This one measures the ability of your liver to eliminate toxins. Many natural health practitioners do this by giving you a caffeine tablet, an aspirin, and two acetaminophen tablets.

Each of these is detoxified by a separate pathway of the liver. Converted into metabolic byproducts, these substances can then be detected through a urine sample.

Accurate diagnosis: Not a simple matter

As you can see, accurately diagnosing this syndrome is not a simple matter. But if you consider that a correct diagnosis may help relieve a variety of unrelated ailments and get you feeling well again, it's certainly well worth the effort.

When you receive your diagnosis, your physician will provide you with a course of treatment. The following chapter includes some of the items he or she will probably touch on with you.

You may want to stay one step ahead and start making some of the right changes in your lifestyle and habits immediately. That's great. Curious and eager to rid your body of this problem? The next chapter is a great beginning.

Chapter 4
Rebalancing the Digestive System

U p until now, you've been learning about the causes of leaky gut syndrome. You've also discovered that diagnosing the problem with any accuracy isn't an easy (or quick) task.

You're also probably realizing how this syndrome, which is seldom spoken of in allopathic medical circles, may be harming your system more than you initially realized.

You're also wondering if anything can be done to improve the situation. Leaky gut syndrome seems, at the very least, a vicious circle you're sentenced to live with.

It also appears to be a very sneaky disorder. It masquerades as any number of other ailments. While you're busy treating it as one condition, it continues to grow worse. But in this chapter, you're about to learn some of the tips, tricks, and techniques to outwit this stealthy health condition.

Indeed, many individuals whose allopathic doctors don't recognize this disorder must live with it. But that isn't necessarily the case. Certainly it doesn't mean you must.

The good news is that leaky gut syndrome can be cured

And the even-better news is that it can be accomplished without the use of harsh, potentially harmful and dangerous medications.

But that means you're completely responsible for the state of your health. Recovering from this disorder is solely in your hands. I've got plenty of confidence in you, though.

I know you'll learn how to change habits — and stick with them — and use some nutritional supplements to help augment the process. You'll dive into repairing your digestive tract and, before you know it, you'll be on the road to recovery.

Here's just one word of warning

You may have been suffering from leaky gut syndrome for some time now — probably longer than you can imagine. Your digestive system certainly won't be healed overnight – and not in a matter of a day or two. But if you're determined to get well, you will.

Listen to your body

Another key to getting well is following your individual needs. Previously, you may have ignored your body when it tried to tell you something was amiss. Or perhaps you've tried to listen, but not understood what it was saying.

Now you're armed with much more information and awareness of the situation than you had before. And you have a fuller understanding of what your true health issues are. This means you'll be much more attuned to the clues your body is sending you. Listen to them carefully.

Patience—Perseverance—Persistence

These three qualities are guaranteed to help you heal from this disorder. And so are the guidelines that are to follow. Before I even talk about the changes in your diet and any nutritional supplements you need to be taking, I've provided you with a few secrets others have used successfully. Not only are they useful for you now, they're just healthy habits to establish.

A quick starter's guide

Even before you begin changing your diet, you can take a simple step. It involves chewing your food. Most of us chew, not only too fast, but also too hard.

Relax when you eat. How many meals have you eaten recently that were hurriedly consumed in a car or downed quickly before you entered into an important meeting? Probably more than you care to admit.

Every doctor tells you the same thing: chewing is the first step to a healthy digestive tract.

I'm going to let you in a secret most people aren't aware of: chewing your food is necessary because it increases the surface area of the food. Doesn't sound like a big deal, does it?

But increasing the surface area means that your digestive system won't have to work so hard. The saliva produced while you chew holds digestive enzymes that actually initiate the process of digestion on both carbohydrates and the fats.

Parotid glands—glands located under your tongue— deliver messages not only to your digestive tract, but to your brain as well. They tell them what to expect. If you don't chew properly, you'll catch them by surprise.

As part of your new lifestyle

You're probably facing many changes in your lifestyle when it comes to your diet — at least if you're seriously tackling this syndrome.

As part of the healing process, there are a few factors you should keep in mind. The first involves any food allergies you may have. Most people with this health condition have a few. Any food allergies or even food sensitivities (which may be even more difficult to detect than allergies) should not be ignored. Indeed, treating these is a major key to healing.

The best advice is to avoid those foods for a minimum of four to six months. If you have numerous food allergies, you may want to seriously consider a rotation diet.

You can take the initial steps through a process called *reseeding the gut.* This is a term Frank Lipman uses in his book called, *Total Renewal: 7 Key Steps to Resilience, Vitality and Long-Term Health.*

While this may sound complicated and difficult, it really isn't. It involves restoring beneficial bacteria and tissues to your body. Beneficial bacteria are often referred to as probiotics.

Unlike antibiotics, which kill the toxic bacteria, probiotics actually provide your body with an abundance of healthy or *friendly* bacteria that keep your system running smoothly and infections and toxins in check.

The dark side of antibiotics

Any number of actions can destroy your system's supply of probiotics, including consuming too much junk food—those nutritionally empty snacks. In addition, healthy bacteria may be destroyed by the use of some medications.

Antibiotics are the obvious cause. While they're obviously beneficial by killing the bacteria causing infections and disease, in the process they also kill off a portion of your friendly bacteria.

And believe it or not, even the use of hormones can destroy healthy bacteria, as can the ingestion of steroids. Now you can see how easily a digestive system can be harmed.

Introducing: The elimination diet

One of the most popular ways of restoring balance is by changing eating habits. Many individuals use versions of what's called the "elimination diet" to deal with food allergies, and especially food sensitivities, which far too often are the underlying cause of leaky gut syndrome.

It's a simple diet in theory; not so simple to execute. The hectic lifestyle of the average American — and no doubt you can attest to this in your daily life — is that there aren't enough hours in the day. Far too often, you probably eat fast food, restaurant take out, and easy-to-prepare packaged foods.

In many ways, this way of eating is nothing more than a coping mechanism. Sometimes it's the only way we can make it through the week. How many of your friends work forty plus hours a week (both Mom and Dad), chauffeur children to dance lessons, soccer and who knows what else? Finding time to make dinner is often an afterthought.

But look at what we as a society are calling nutritious fare. Good grief, we have "processed cheese food" slices that are supposed to take the place of real cheese, shakes at fast food restaurants that don't label themselves as milkshakes (so exactly what are they made of?), and some taco meat that isn't 100 percent beef.

Is it any wonder your digestive system is rebelling?

Kick processed foods to the curb

As part of an elimination diet, these foods have to be the first to be... well, eliminated. Chockfull of additives and unnatural colorings, they're very often the worst offenders.

You'll also be asked on any elimination diet to forgo refined sugar, refined white flour, and grains containing gluten. These, too, can play havoc with your digestive system.

This is not to say you can never eat any of these foods again. But you'll add foods back into your system slowly, most likely one food at a time. Then you check your body's response.

This method of food testing serves a two-fold process. First, by eliminating many of the worst offenders for a minimum of a month, you're allowing your body to rebalance. In that time, you'll be supplying it with many of the nutrients and probiotics to restore a proper bacteria-flora ratio.

It also allows you to provide your body many of the proper nutrients that the packaged, processed, and fast foods don't have. Between these two aspects, you'll begin to feel better.

Withdrawal symptoms

Here's a word of warning. You may begin to feel worse before you feel better. Your body has grown dependent on many of these foods — especially refined sugar.

So withholding these foods from your system may produce temporary adverse reactions. Once you get past these symptoms, however, you'll experience all the benefits that are promised through this method.

As mentioned, most people discover that one month of abstinence from these offenders is enough to rebalance and rebuild. For some individuals, though, it may take up to three months before any definitive results can be seen.

So exactly what foods are we talking about? It depends on the diet you've chosen. But all versions of this diet are very similar. You'll want to concentrate on eating fresh fruits and vegetables as much as possible.

When you eat proteins and meats, go light on the beef and red meat. If at all possible think organic meats and free- range chickens. Not only are these foods healthier for you, but you'll discover that they have a distinctly better taste than what you've been eating.

While I won't go into any details about a specific diet in this chapter, the appendix has a sample of a three-phase elimination diet that may give you some idea about how this works.

Many individuals may find jumping into one of these diets daunting. Others may just find it impossible to go "cold turkey" from packaged and processed foods.

If you're one of these people, then you can take "baby steps" to start the process in motion. Once you start doing this, you may decide that you can wean yourself off the salt-laden packaged and frozen foods stuffed with artificial additives. Believe me, any step you take toward mending your diet will help.

The great balancing act of bacteria

One of the hallmark symptoms of leaky gut syndrome is the predominance of bad bacteria over good flora. In rebalancing your imbalance, you'll probably want to enlist the aid of your personal physician or a natural healthcare provider.

He or she can offer any number of natural methods to facilitate this. The most effective of these include using garlic, oil of oregano capsules, grapefruit seed extract, mathake tea, berberine, capryllic acid, pau d'arco, and tanalbit.

In addition, you'll want to begin treating the presence of any Candida yeast infection. This fungus actually responds well to not only dietary changes, but to treatment with natural substances.

Follow a few simple guidelines

You'll also want to follow a few simple guidelines. The most imperative steps are to eat a low-carbohydrate diet and avoid sugar, alcohol, and vinegar.

You'll also want to include the use of a high-quality probiotic product. A probiotic is an organism that can be most easily described as the friendly flora in your intestines. And a good one contains millions of live bacteria. Once you "reinforce" your system, the added flora not only help to reestablish your balance, but actually stop the growth of the bad bacteria as well.

What's more, the addition of probiotics goes a long way toward boosting your immune system.

One of the aspects of Candida is their innate instinct of survival. You may discover that even after you diligently treat your Candida infections with probiotics, some yeast is still stubbornly clinging to you. In order to clear your system thoroughly, you may have to use one or more alternative methods to ensure the infection is gone.

Another word of caution: as you treat your fungal infection, it may worsen. Don't panic.

Consider the rotation diet

This is especially good advice if you suffer from multiple food allergies. The rotation diet is a good method for keeping your food allergies under control. And it might be easier than the elimination diet to start for some people. Basically, you eat biologically related foods on the same day. Then you wait a minimum of four days before you eat them again.

So how does this help you? For starters, it stops the continuation of any development of new food allergies. While there are some foods that are more widely known to trigger an allergic reaction, just about any food, if eaten too often, can prompt an allergy. This is especially true if you already are prone to them, or if you have leaky gut syndrome.

Using this diet, you can actually eat the foods you have a mild or borderline reaction to, while reducing the symptoms. Some individuals prefer to test drive the rotation diet before they jump into an elimination diet.

While the standard rotation diet usually advises a four-day rotation plan, you may find that a longer period is necessary for some foods. The most common foods which trigger allergies include wheat, corn, citrus fruits, legumes, and cow's milk.

Discover the benefits of FOS foods

If you haven't heard of FOS foods, you're not alone. Most people are totally unaware of these foods and of FOS in particular.

But you may have a genuine interest in it soon, once you learn how it can help rebalance your digestive system and alleviate the symptoms of leaky gut syndrome.

FOS stands for an excruciatingly long word, *fructooligosaccharide*. This is a specialized type of sugar molecule which actually increases the growth of flora — especially lactobacillus, an especially friendly flora.

The foods rich in this molecule include:

- Asparagus

- Bananas

- Barley

- Onions

- Fruit

- Leeks

- Jerusalem artichoke

- Garlic

- Burdock

- Chicory

- Wheat

- Soybeans

Increase your consumption of these foods and you'll be helping to rebalance your digestive system.

Let's talk fruits and vegetables in general

Sure, your mother probably had this talk with you already as she impressed upon you the importance of fruits and vegetables in your diet. But this time we're approaching the issue from a slightly different angle.

There exists good scientific reasoning — and research — behind this time-honored advice. These foods are richly endowed with substances called *antioxidants*. No doubt you've head of them. They're credited with helping to keep you from developing such conditions as dangerous as heart disease and cancer. Antioxidants also help to boost your immune system.

But, beyond that, as a person who suffers with leaky gut syndrome, these healing substances may have even more meaning for you.

First, do you really know what antioxidants are and how they work in your system? To truly appreciate their importance, you need to understand what they do.

Hooray for antioxidants

Every day, untold numbers of cells are damaged by specific molecules known as free radicals. Sometimes you'll hear these referred to as "reactive oxygen species," or ROS.

Your body produces these substances naturally as a response to metabolism. But they are also produced in other ways. They grow quickly when you consume alcohol and when you're exposed to cigarettes, radiation, drugs, and rancid oil.

But that's not the only way they grow — and grow rapidly. Exposure to the sun also causes an increase in their growth rate and subjects your body to stress.

These free radicals are basically unstable molecules searching for stability. They seek out electrons and snatch them for themselves. And they don't care where they get them.

These harmful substances usually target your cell and mitochondrial membranes, as well as your nervous system. They can adversely affect your enzymes, too. This is particularly dangerous because enzymes are charged with ensuring healthy cellular function.

But that's not all. They also have the potential to damage your DNA, which is the structure determining the way in which your cells replicate.

While this occurs in everyone, the presence of free radicals is even more dangerous once your intestinal tract is injured. At this point, they occur in such vast numbers that your system can't control them.

Some experts claim that one free radical can potentially adversely affect one million cells. The exact amount of damage created, though, depends on the ability of your body to recognize what's happening to it — and then, of course, the availability of antioxidant nutrients to combat them.

Working in concert

This is where antioxidants play a key role. There are different types of antioxidants, and each specific type is assigned individual tasks that complement the others. To be effective, they must be used as a group. Antioxidants are found in many fruits and vegetables, so it's really no surprise that so many health experts recommend these foods.

By now, you're probably beginning to get a sense of how your body works in harmony with the foods you provide it to keep it running in top form.

In addition to fruits and vegetables, rich sources of antioxidants include nuts and seeds. The truth of the matter is that most foods, if eaten in their natural state, have active antioxidants. Once we process these foods by freezing them or using them in packaged and processed foods, we kill their effectiveness.

Have you cleansed your system lately?

And this is exactly the reason why some specialists who treat leaky gut syndrome recommend a fruit and vegetable cleansing. It's not only an effective method of detoxification, but it's also gentle on your system.

Before we talk about this cleanse, let me caution you that any change in diet — especially one which relies on a specific genre of foods exclusively — should be cleared with your personal physician.

He or she has a working knowledge of what kind of changes your body can handle.

In a nutshell, the fruit and vegetable cleanse is exactly what it sounds like. You eat only fresh fruits and vegetables for seven to ten days. You can also use olive and canola oils as condiments during this time.

Add fresh fruit and vegetable juices after ten days. These are incredibly powerful and concentrated sources of nutrients which your body can use easily. Juices also have the advantage of being able to enhance detoxification pathways.

As in any cleansing regimen, you may experience discomfort the first several days. Many individuals report they develop headaches. This symptom could occur for any number of reasons, including sugar or caffeine withdrawal.

But don't let that discourage you. The simple fact that you're experiencing withdrawal symptoms indicates that the cleansing is working. Toxins are being flushed out of your system.

Attacking withdrawal symptoms easily

One effective way to deal with withdrawal symptoms is to drink water, diluted fruit juices, and decaffeinated herbal teas. This hastens the elimination of toxins.

Other individuals say they develop a rash or pimples. This is merely another indicator that the cleansing process is working. These symptoms mean that toxins are being eliminated through your skin. You can ease the situation through steam baths, saunas, and even massaging your skin with a loofa or a soft dry brush.

Yet others discover they develop constipation. You may take a fiber supplement to help. You might also discover that psyllium seeds or freshly ground flaxseeds help. Start with one teaspoon of either of these in water then drink quickly before it turns into a gel.

These are simply basic guidelines to get you started on adjusting your diet to help heal your health condition. It's easy enough to start with small steps. Don't discount the effectiveness of taking any step — no matter how small. If continued and you add steps as you go along, you'll discover a whole new healthy you.

While you're adjusting your diet, you may also want to augment and heighten the effects by taking nutritional supplements. They can help add a punch to your other efforts.

Curious about which are the best? Turn to the next chapter. I'll give you some ideas about the best supplements to get you started.

Chapter 5
Rebalancing with Nutritional Supplements

You've already learned the importance of transforming your diet from artificial to fresh. Perhaps you've even embarked on a few steps toward that goal. Good for you. But, don't stop there. There are other steps you can take to augment these changes.

They come in the form of nutritional and dietary supplements. While the best form of getting your vitamins, minerals, and antioxidants is obviously through whole, fresh foods, the imbalance in your system may demand additional help.

That's where these amazing nutritional boosts come in. They may give you just the right amount of the needed building blocks to help battle an unhealthy condition that's been allowed to sit in your digestive system for too long.

So what types of nutritional supplements am I talking about? This chapter provides you with a variety from which to choose. You're bound to find at least one that helps you in curing your leaky gut syndrome.

Health food stores have the largest selection of nutritional supplements and sales clerks can often offer helpful information.

Vitamins and minerals: Vitamin A

Vitamin A is an essential nutrient for a healthy gastrointestinal tract. Vitamin A triggers the production of protective antibodies known as SigA. Additionally, this familiar nutrient also aids in the maintenance of your intestinal mucosa. An added benefit is its ability to ease inflammation.

The availability of various forms of vitamin A are plentiful from health food stores, vitamin shops, and even grocery stores. But you may want to search for a specific form of this essential health building block. It's called an *emulsion*. It'll cost a little more, but it's probably the most effective form. It literally coats the intestinal mucosa, working its way to all the most crucial areas. And it can be taken without any fear of adverse side effects in servings of 20,000 to 25,000 IU daily.

It's a family affair: vitamin B complex

It truly is a family affair when it comes to the B-complex of vitamins. And because of the dysbiosis that is a natural part of leaky gut syndrome, the family is under attack.

But it's B-12 that's especially threatened by this imbalance of bacteria in your small intestines. And for this reason, you may develop — in addition to your leaky gut problems — pernicious anemia. Pernicious anemia occurs when your body is lacking in Vitamin B-12, even though it's apparently receiving an adequate supply through dietary sources and supplementation.

That's not surprising with leaky gut. Its hallmark symptom, as we've said many times, is the blocking of the absorption of many nutrients.

For the average person, a vitamin B-12 deficiency is extremely rare. The body stores several years' worth ensuring you stay healthy. But for those with leaky gut, your body can't access the stores and the nutrient is of no use.

Before supplementing your system with this vitamin, you might want to ask your doctor to run simple blood tests to see if you're low in B-12. Then he or she can find the proper way to help you rebuild your system.

It's important you do this because, along with the rest of the nutrient family, B-12 is essential in the proper functioning of your nervous system.

Vitamin C's potent antioxidant abilities

If there were ever a "superhero" of the vitamin world, it would be vitamin C. It has long been known as an effective immune booster. Millions of people take it religiously during cold and flu season.

There are two excellent reasons why it's a supplement worth taking if you suffer from this disorder. Leaky gut syndrome, as we noted earlier, is partially caused by the presence of free radicals in your system. So far, the scientific community has discovered that antioxidants are the most effective way to neutralize the damaging effects of these scavenger molecules. And vitamin C is a potent antioxidant.

But more than that, the immune-boosting power of this vitamin can help heal this disorder as well.

Some health experts recommend as much as 4,500 mg of vitamin C daily. Start taking this supplement slowly, perhaps as little as 500 to 1,000 mg daily. See how you feel. Sometimes taking large amounts of vitamin C can backfire on you and cause digestive issues.

Don't underrate vitamin E

Another known powerful antioxidant, vitamin E, probably ranks second only to vitamin C in its usefulness. Its area of specialty as an antioxidant is healing tissues from free-radical damage. Like vitamin C, it also possesses incredible immune-boosting powers.

Even though you may be eating all the right foods, especially if you've embarked on your elimination diet, consider supplementing your diet with this powerful source of healing.

According to the Office of Dietary Supplements, an adult can safely take 1,000 mg a day. You may want to start off slowly, though, so your body can adjust to the nutrient.

What about magnesium?

This trace mineral merits a second look if you suffer from leaky gut syndrome, according to recently released research. It seems that those who suffer from this condition and from one of the consequential disorders it triggers — fibromyalgia — appear to be prone to a deficiency of magnesium.

This deficiency occurs, in part, when your intestinal walls become inflamed, damaging many of the carrier proteins necessary for the transportation of this mineral.

Since the problem isn't merely a matter of consumption, but absorption, you may be suffering from a lack of magnesium, even though you're eating foods abundant in the nutrient. That's why it's vital that the inflammation is treated as quickly as possible.

You can safely take a maximum of 350 mg of magnesium daily.

It's time to think... zinc

This mineral is rapidly being recognized as a healing substance. It's perfect specifically for cells with a rapid turnover, just like those of the small intestine mucosa. Being replaced at the rate of approximately every four days, these cells require zinc to strengthen the integrity of the intestinal lining.

Recent research reveals that zinc supplementation may ease or heal Crohn's disease as well.

Taking zinc supplements, even if your diet is rich in foods abundant in this mineral, is a good idea. Your body uses zinc at an amazing rate, so it may be difficult to keep up with its depletion. It's not surprising that research performed recently by Dr. Keith Eaton, working for an organization called Biolab based in London, uncovered that zinc is the most common nutritional deficiency among leaky gut syndrome sufferers.

So how much do I need?

Most natural health experts recommend servings between 50 to 80 mg daily. This range is large enough, they say, to rebalance any deficiency of zinc. While usually more is better, they also advise not to take more than 100 mg a day.

This level of supplementation helps bolster your immune system. But any serving exceeding this actually has an adverse effect on your immune system.

Healthcare professionals also recommend taking zinc in conjunction with copper. For every 15 mg of zinc you take, you should take 1 mg of copper. Taking zinc supplements can actually deplete your copper level.

Supplements with nutraceuticals to help heal leaky gut

Wikipedia describes a nutraceutical as a product isolated or purified from foods that is demonstrated to have a physiological benefit or provide protection against chronic disease.

Brenda Watson, CNC in her book, "The Road to Perfect Health: Balance your Gut, Heal Your Body," describes the importance of taking supplements with nutraceuticals to control leaky gut and help heal the body.

Leaky gut syndrome is a major part of the gut connection to so many health conditions that affect the rest of the body. I cannot stress enough the importance of rebuilding the gut lining. The gut lining needs to be intact so that the beneficial bacteria can adhere to it properly. This creates the proper defense against invading pathogens and toxins. If this gut protection system is not in place, chronic and recurrent health conditions will develop.

Reducing toxic exposure is of prime importance in preventing and reversing leaky gut syndrome. Both exotoxins (which come from the outside environment) and endotoxins (which are produced inside the body by bacteria and poor digestive conditions) can contribute to a leaky gut. Eliminating these toxins, maintaining regular elimination and healing the intestinal lining are key steps in healing a leaky gut.

...nutraceuticals along with other traditionally used supplements can provide powerful support for the organs and organ systems responsible for filtering and eliminating toxins from the body and restoring vibrant health and energy...

The most critical: glutamine

L-glutamine is probably the most important amino acid in the maintenance of both the structure and the function of the intestine, and is essential for a healthy metabolism. It can be acquired naturally through many high-protein foods.

It's also vital for you, as one who suffers from leaky gut syndrome, for another reason as well. It's the body's "preferred fuel" for the cells which line the mucosa of your small intestine. These particular cells use glutamine directly rather than waiting for the bloodstream to deliver them.

Another task assigned to this amino acid is the prevention of the translocation of bacteria from the gut into the bloodstream — a vital aspect to healing leaky gut syndrome.

For these reasons, your body needs a generous quantity of glutamine for the repair and maintenance of a healthy small intestinal lining.

The foods rich in this substance include beans, beef, beats, cabbage, chicken, dairy products and fish.

How to obtain additional glutamine

Considering its overarching importance in the health of those who suffer with leaky gut syndrome, you may want to seriously consider taking a glutamine supplement. To be most effective the supplement should be combined with gamma oryzanol (a mixture of antioxidant compounds) and is best taken in powder form.

I've included a list of other supplements also found to be effective in treating leaky gut:

Helpful:

- **Total Body Cleanse (herb formula)**

Encourages elimination and detoxification.

- **Bentonite clay/Glucomannan/**

   Charcoal Formula

Helps absorb toxins from the GI tract.

- **Antioxidant Supplement**

Protects tissue from damage.

• High Potency multi-vitamin/mineral

For overall good health.

For Daily Maintenance:

• L-Glutamine Powder with Gamma Oryzanol

Helps repair the intestinal lining, reducing permeability and reducing severe reactions to foods.

• Digestive Enzymes

Helps digest and absorb nutrients from food.

• Probiotics

Numerous benefits to intestinal health—helps reduce permeability and inflammation.

• Omega-3 Fatty Acids

Helps restore moisture to the intestinal tract. Provides lubrication.

• Fiber

Helps produce healthy bacteria levels and good elimination

Choose your nutritional supplements carefully. I use Renew Life supplements because the company is targeted specifically to digestive health. I know there are other good companies as well.

One of the steps I took, as a part of my leaky gut regimen, was to start taking a digestive enzyme with each meal, which helps me digest and absorb nutrients from food. This one change alone has made a tremendous impact on my wellbeing.

You should not only inform your healthcare provider that you're taking these supplements, but ask for advice. He or she knows your specific symptoms and perhaps has run blood tests that may shed light on what nutrients you're deficient in.

Working hand in hand with a physician who understands leaky gut syndrome is the best avenue you can choose.

Another method of supplementing your diet and restoring balance is through the use of herbal supplements. Many of these plants are packed with vitamins, minerals and phytonutrients that can enhance your health.

The following chapter describes just a few of the very best herbs for leaky gut syndrome.

Chapter 6
Rebalancing With Herbs

Healing with herbs is an old and honored tradition and potentially an effective way to improve your health. A wide variety of cultures have turned to plants to help them restore health.

It may surprise you to learn that many of the prescription medications that so many of us depend on today were originally taken from plants. Aspirin and some heart medications are only two prime examples.

So it only makes sense that to help heal your leaky gut syndrome, you may want to turn to these amazing nutritional natural aids.

Before you embark on any supplementation program, be sure you consult with your personal physician. Tell her or him what you're planning to take to ensure there are no conflicts with any prescription medications you're taking.

But you may also want to go one step beyond that. Before deciding on a herbal regimen, consider consulting a professional herbalist. A herbalist has spent years studying herbs through an accredited school. He or she will be able to help you pinpoint exactly what will help your symptoms and condition.

Of course, once you consult an herbalist, you may end up with a list of suggestions. In the meantime, here are some suggestions to get you thinking about what's possible.

Slippery elm for leaky gut

If you're at all familiar with herbal remedies, then you might already know something about the herb slippery elm. For more than 100 years, professional herbalists have relied on this plant as a healing salve for wounds, burns, skin inflammation, boils, ulcers... need I go on?

It also happens to be an effective agent when taken internally as well. In addition to its ability to treat coughs, sore throats, and diarrhea, this versatile herb can also help remedy stomach problems.

Why?

Slippery elm possesses a mucilage. Mucilage is a substance which turns to gel when mixed with water. It forms a coat and soothes your mouth, throat, stomach, and intestines.

But that's not all. This amazing herb also contains an abundance of antioxidants. We've already established that antioxidants can help reduce free radicals, which in turn aids in the cure of leaky gut. In particular, this herb relieves inflammatory infections in the bowel, according to the herbalists.

It also triggers reflux stimulation of the nerve endings in your gastrointestinal tract, which eventually lead to an increase in mucus secretion. That's a good thing. This increase in production protects your gastrointestinal tract from such disorders as ulcers and acidity.

In essence, slippery elm soothes and calms an inflamed and damaged gut lining. Specifically, it's this soothing action which eventually allows the antioxidants to perform their tasks.

Peppermint tea, anyone?

Think about it for an even a moment and you'll agree that peppermint tea seems to be a natural choice in helping to alleviate your leaky gut. And that's because herbalists have been using it for a variety of stomach problems and any other number of disorders for... well, it seems like forever.

This remarkable drink has calming and numbing powers. But beyond that, peppermint tea kills certain kinds of bacteria. Even research is now showing that it is a credible defense against indigestion and irritable bowel syndrome.

When you drink this tea, the ingredients in this herb calm the stomach and promote the flow of bile, a needed ingredient in the digestion of fats. This enables food to pass through the stomach more quickly.

How to use peppermint tea

If you prepare this brew yourself using peppermint you've grown in your herb garden, use the dried leaves of the plant. Prepare your tea by steeping one teaspoon of · the dried leaves in a cup of boiling water for approximately 10 minutes.

Then strain and cool the mixture. For the best results, drink it four or five times a day between meals.

However, growing your own peppermint is not necessary because this tea is widely available. You can also purchase enteric-coated capsules. These are specially coated so the capsule may pass through the stomach into the intestine.

Most herbal specialists recommend one or two capsules taken at least two times a day. Some say the optimum serving is two capsules three times daily. This latter recommendation is especially pertinent if you have irritable bowel syndrome.

The versatility of chamomile tea

Chamomile tea is another well-known and greatly used tea that may benefit you. This tea is already considered a calming and relaxing agent; many individuals drink it as part of their nightly bedtime ritual.

Additionally, this tea is credited with strong antispasmodic and anti-inflammatory ingredients, which can be effective in the treatment of stomach problems and intestinal cramps.

It's a recommended remedy for the cramping and pain of the bowels associated with irritable bowel syndrome.

Additionally, chamomile tea helps with the excessive gas and bloating of the intestines.

All you may need to remedy this, in fact, is a single cup of chamomile tea daily. That's certainly easy enough.

This tea can be purchased practically anywhere. It's not only available in health food stores and vitamin shops, but it can be found commercially in just about any grocery store.

No, marshmallow root has nothing to do with s'mores

While the herb marshmallow root has nothing to do with that campfire treat s'mores, it has everything to do with soothing the irritated mucous membranes of your upper respiratory tract and your digestive tract.

And that means it may be just the supplement you're looking for to help heal leaky gut syndrome. Don't let the name fool you. Marshmallow root — many times referred to as "mallow" — has a healing history that literally extends thousands of years in the past. Talk about being tested by time.

This root is extremely effective in helping almost all problems related to the inflammation of your digestive tract. It could be just the remedy that can help you overcome leaky gut.

While it may be difficult to find this supplement at your local grocery store, you should have no trouble finding it at health food stores and vitamin shops. And of course, if you can't find it any place else, you can always purchase it online.

Herbs that eliminate parasites

We talked earlier about the presence of parasites in many individuals who suffer with leaky gut syndrome. There is a combination of three herbal tinctures you may want to take that can help you rid your body of the parasites.

One of the advantages of this healing blend is its effectiveness on more than 100 different types of parasites. Using the proper serving, it kills not only the adult parasites but the eggs as well. The tinctures are black walnut green, wormwood, and cloves.

When I talk about the black walnut green tincture, I'm referring to the use of the green hull that surrounds the nut of the black walnut tree. According to many herbalists, its ability to kill parasites is near miraculous. It's important that the hull is used while it is green. Once it turns black, it loses its active ingredients.

In many instances, the black walnut supplements found in vitamin shops and health food stores are made with the hull after it has turned black. You may want to work closely with a professional licensed herbalist in order to ensure your black walnut tincture is effective.

The walnut and wormwood are the herbs that effectively kill off the adult parasites, while the third herb, the cloves tincture, kills the eggs.

Echinacea and the elimination of leaky gut

If you're not familiar with echinacea, you're in for a pleasant surprise.

Echinacea is one of the most widely used herbs in this country, and with good reason. Its history goes back at least 400 years. Native Americans used it to treat infections and wounds. In fact, you'll discover that this amazingly versatile herb is probably the closest you'll find to an "all-purpose" herb.

Used worldwide, there were diverse reasons for people to reach out to this plant. Uses include treating scarlet fever, malaria, blood poisoning, and even diphtheria.

Echinacea probably reached its peak in popularity in the 18th and 19th centuries. With the advent of prescription antibiotics, it quickly faded from public use. But now it's making a stunning resurgence as people discover the dangers of using harsh medications.

Its popularity is not surprising since research confirms its effectiveness. Several studies reveal that its active ingredients improve the immune system, reduce inflammation, and possess antioxidant qualities.

For many herbalists, echinacea is the first choice in the treatment of Candida as well as several other infections.

Many individuals find using echinacea, the well-established herb that's a natural antibiotic, helps them in avoiding the overuse of prescription antibiotics. Instead of visiting their doctor and filling a prescription, they reach for this herb.

Of course, this herb won't work for all infections, but it helps those who tend to overuse or even abuse antibiotic medications.

Now that I have it, what do I do with it?

For the most part, herbalists suggest that you take echinacea three times daily for seven to 10 days in order to ensure that you receive its full antibiotic benefits.

You also have the choice of using it in a number of forms. If you're lucky enough to have some fresh herbs, you'll want to dry the root or the plant itself and use it as a tea. For this purpose, you'll need one to two grams.

If you're using a standardized tincture extract, you'll need 2 to 3 ml of the liquid. As a powdered extract, you'll need 300 mg of the standardized powder.

How popular is the herb? Actually, if there's such a thing as being too popular, then echinacea is it. It's being used at such an incredible rate that it's currently overharvested. It's in danger of become an endangered species.

Another shining star: goldenseal

Another favorite of herbalists in the treatment of leaky gut is goldenseal, an herb that, like echinacea has a legendary reputation when it comes to digestive issues.

Goldenseal has just the right combination of abilities that can make it an invaluable dietary supplement if you're troubled with a leaky gut. It not only works quickly on digestive issues, but it also has antibacterial traits. In a nutshell, it's a natural antibiotic.

More often than not, this herb is paired with echinacea to create a powerful supplement that not only helps the digestive tract, but bolsters your immune system as well.

Goldenseal is available just about everywhere — in health food stores, vitamin shops, and even grocery stores. You have your choice in taking the tablet form or the capsule variety.

Pau d'arco

You may not have heard of Pau d'arco, a plant native to South America. On that continent, its history of use is wide ranging. It's been used to control pain, keep arthritis at bay and to treat inflammation.

Pau d'arco is often used to treat candida infections and any number of bacterial infections. You're already well aware that candida is a disorder that goes hand-in-hand with leaky gut. This herb also attacks another symptom of leaky gut — the presence of parasites.

If you plan on taking Pau d'arco, you have your choice in what form you take. From tablets to dried bark teas and tinctures, you can find any of these at health food and vitamin shops. But you may also want to visit a professional herbalist to help you get a tailor-made formula to meet your unique needs.

The most common serving is 300 to 500 mg in capsule form three times a day. If you're using a tincture, you'll use between ½ to 1 ml two to three times daily.

In this book, we've reviewed many of the ways to get your body healthy through diet and supplementation — both nutritional and herbal.

Another cause of leaky gut syndrome

But what about that other cause and major aggravator of leaky gut syndrome—stress? It's everywhere—more than two-thirds of Americans say they are likely to seek help for stress. Fifty-four percent of Americans are concerned about the level of stress in their everyday lives. Fifty-five percent of people say their stress is caused by not having enough time to do the things they need to do. I'm guessing you probably fall somewhere within this statistical framework. At work, at home, at school, even in your daily commute.

Is there anything that can be done to eliminate stress?

You can't eliminate stress from your body, but you can learn how to manage it intelligently. The following chapter gives you some clues on how to do just that.

Chapter 7
On the Path to Good Health: Stress Management and Beyond

Stress—the final frontier. Well, maybe not. But it certainly is one of the ongoing problems of the twenty-first century. Today, you're probably feeling the stress more than ever. Stress has become an unspoken but omnipresent fact of life.

But more than that, stress has become one of the causes of ill health. Did you know that the World Health Organization has listed on-the-job stress as one of the top ten reasons for poor health? In fact, one in three adults suffer from moderate to extreme stress. That's one third of the population.

Not one of us spends a day without encountering some type of stressful situation. It can be work-induced, or caused by a concern such as paying bills, or a super-tight schedule. Stress is unavoidable.

Many insist stress is a good thing. In moderation, it certainly is. It motivates us to work harder, to meet goals we might not have accomplished otherwise. And there are those people who say they work best under stress.

It certainly served our ancestors well. The caveman experienced stress when confronted with dangers such as the presence of a woolly mammoth. Once the stress mechanism kicked in, it gave our prehistoric ancestor the strength and energy either to fight the large creature or to run from it.

But in prehistoric times, our ancient ancestors didn't deal with stress on a daily or even hourly basis, as we do today. They encountered stress far less often. The caveman's reaction to stress actually was a life-saving mechanism instead of the health-draining reaction it has become.

Reacting to stress

Today, our reaction to tense situations, to the pressures of work, home, money, or anything else, is reflected in our physical well-being. That's right — your reaction to the pressures of daily life has a direct bearing on your physical body.

In fact, how you choose to react to stress affects the status of your health. For starters, it's well known that prolonged exposure to pressures can actually lower your immune system.

The truth of the matter is that, if you allow it, stress can take a devastating toll on your body. Your reaction to stress may be one of the causes of leaky gut syndrome.

Let's face it, we can't avoid stress. Regardless of how hard we try (or how stressed out we get trying to avoid stress), it's a part of our lives. This means you have to learn how to live with it. And I'm not talking about just giving in to the tension. I'm speaking about how to meet it and beat it and keep your cool — and your health.

Let me go one step further. Studies reveal that taking specific steps — beginning certain programs — actually produce physical and chemical changes in your body that help you to feel better.

When do I start my stress-reduction program?

Soon actually. But first, you need to do a thorough examination of your life to see how stress is affecting you.

Trust me. There are symptoms that clue you in to this, but you have to be able to recognize them. Perhaps you're experiencing them but not realizing the cause. Leaky gut syndrome is a perfect example. Even if you treat it nutritionally, you may find it recurs if stress is clogging your life.

Signs, signs… everywhere are signs

Your reaction to stress differs from your co-worker's. It differs from how your spouse may react. How you react is a very personal, very individualized response. The physical symptoms you develop may not be the same as everyone else's.

But, guaranteed, there is a set of signs that indicate the situation is affecting your body. I've listed some of them here.

Examine your feelings. Are you feeling anxious, irritable, or fearful? Are you experiencing mood swings you don't understand? Even feeling unexplained embarrassment can all be attributed to an emotional response to stress.

Carefully review what you're thinking. It's true. When you're "stressed-out," it's reflected in your thoughts. You may find you're more critical of yourself, or you may have noticed you just can't concentrate.

Are you having trouble making decisions? Or perhaps you've noticed you're forgetful. Other signs that stress may be harming you physically (and mentally) include a preoccupation with the future, repeating the same thoughts over and over, and the constant fear of failure.

Study your behavior. If you're reacting poorly to stress, it definitely will reveal itself in your behavior. Do you find yourself crying for no apparent reason, or over small, trivial things? Have you noticed a change in your normal eating habits — either eating more or suddenly having no appetite?

Are you suddenly short-tempered with friends or family members? This is usually one of the first signs that you're not handling stress very well.

Some people deal with stress by turning to alcohol. Has there been a change in the amount you drink in a day? You may also find you're taking up cigarette smoking again, or if you've never quit, you're smoking more than usual.

But there are other small signs, like nervous laughter or teeth grinding or jaw clenching. And others find when stress is adversely affecting them they actually are more accident prone.

Symptoms

Now, let's look at some of the physical symptoms of a stressed-out body. We already recognize that stress can ultimately create or at least worsen leaky gut syndrome. But there are many other signals:

- Sleep problems

- Tight muscles

- Headaches

- Unexplained fatigue

- Cold or sweaty hands

- Neck or back problems

- Stomach distress

- Rapid breathing

- Pounding of the heart

- Dry mouth

And this list only touches the tip of the iceberg. But even from this list, you can see how integrated your emotional and physical health is.

By now you probably realize that since you can't avoid it, you need to learn how to manage stress intelligently.

You may not know where to begin. Start with small simple steps and I guarantee you'll eventually feel it in a big way.

Before I talk about long-term solutions such as yoga, exercise and meditation, here are few steps you can take immediately to help lower your stress level.

Take a long, deep breath...

Yes, it really can be that simple. When you're face-to-face with a stressful situation, one of the first physical signs is shallow breathing. Ironically, this response only creates more stress.

But you can outwit this response by calling a quick time out to do a review of your body. Scan for any possible physical tension. In addition to that shallow breathing, do you have a tight chest? Some individuals actually hold their breath without even knowing it.

Shallow breathing results in a decreased supply of oxygen in your bloodstream and that eventually leads to muscle tension. But that's only the beginning. The next reaction is usually the appearance of a headache. At the very least, you begin to feel even more anxious.

Instead of allowing this chain of events to run its course, you can stop it dead in its tracks... with some practice. Take a minute — yes, I mean 60 seconds — to slow down and breathe deeply.

Inhale through your nose. Exhale through your mouth. Inhale enough breath that your lower abdomen rises and falls. Exhale slowly as you count to 10.

The first time you attempt this you may think it's not working. But this is a wonderful technique, and it's a technique you can learn how to do. Practice it. You'll see how effective it can be.

Practice time management

How much of your day is running from appointment to appointment, eating on the run, and then rushing home in the evening to experience the same habits only with different destinations and purposes?

The truth of the matter is that over-committing is one of the major causes of stress. Instead of throwing up your hands, explaining "That's just how life is," try to manage your time.

No, it won't be easy. In fact, it may take you several attempts to master this. You may have to make some adjustments or even eliminate one or two items from your schedule sometimes. But aren't these small adjustments worth your good health?

Plan ahead. I know it's not as easy as it sounds. But, indeed, it can be done. Start by making a *reasonable* schedule for the day ahead. Also include time in your schedule for stress-reduction exercises.

Many people try to take care of all their needs at once. This futile attempt, a super-multi-tasking if you will, usually results in nothing getting accomplished. You only end up frustrated because another day has passed. You feel — and perhaps rightly so — as if you've accomplished nothing important.

But yet, you continue to function this way. Instead, try a different approach. Make a list (yes, I know you've done this before, but bear with me) of all the tasks that face you for that day.

One task at a time

Only attempt one item at a time. Let me repeat that. *Only tackle one job at a time.* Once you've completed it, check it off your list. Then *and only then* allow yourself to start the second item.

List the items according to their importance. Try to discern priorities. Perform the most important activities first. Don't procrastinate. We all have different reasons for putting certain tasks off. We either dread performing them, or we dread who we have to interact with. Push all those fears aside and just get it over with.

In fact, many of the most efficient people get the most painful tasks out of the way as soon as possible. In that way, they actually get them done and don't have time to… stress about it. And, most importantly, the tasks don't linger on to the next day.

The key to success is not to over schedule yourself or overburden yourself with a list that's impossible to finish. You may be tempted to schedule meetings back to back with little if any time in between. Don't do that. Be liberal in your estimation of certain events and meetings. That way you're not running behind, stressed because you're late for the next event.

Don't isolate yourself. To accomplish some tasks, you certainly need time alone. As a writer, I realize this. I can't share this task with anyone else. I'm sitting alone now, as I write this book. But, I don't spend all my time alone. That's not healthy.

Seek out others

After a certain point you need to walk away from what you're doing. This is true if you've barricaded yourself in your office trying to make a deadline. Even when working against this type of stress, you need to take an occasional break.

Walk to the lunchroom to talk so someone. Visit with the person who has the office next to you. Go down the hall to talk with the receptionist. Keep in touch with others.

Many independent contractors working from home take a day or several hours out of the day to work at a coffee shop or library. This is a healthy habit. It keeps them connected with others.

Talk

This suggestion is a corollary to the last one. One of the reasons for stress is the inability to talk to anyone about your work… your concerns… your problems. Even talking about the events of your daily life helps to relieve stress.

Or perhaps you'd feel more comfortable, at least at the beginning, with writing your concerns out. Just putting your problems or your decisions on paper can assist in such a way that an answer pops into your head.

Don't forget to laugh

No, this isn't included as an afterthought. Maybe the Reader's Digest editorial department has been right all along with their column, "Laughter is the Best Medicine." If it's not the best medicine, it certainly ranks high up there with the top two or three.

No matter what happens, try to keep your sense of humor. Learn how not to take yourself too seriously. And above all, learn how to laugh at yourself.

The one-minute vacation

Never heard of it? It's about time you do. Take a moment to close your eyes. Imagine a place where you feel relaxed. Now, take note of all the details of this location. Imagine not only the physical attributes (is it a beach?) but try to imagine smells, feel the temperature, listen for the sounds that would be there.

This isn't just some random use of your imagination. Research now shows that visualizing a tranquil scene can actually lift you from your stressful situation.

Can't do this on your own? You may want to purchase a CD of guided imagery exercises. There are also CDs for stress relief, relaxation, good health and dozens of other recordings. You can get free samples, so you can try them and see if they're a good fit for you.

Another way to go

Some companies make software that provides affirmation files (which create a positive mindset) in any subject matter you like—like stress relief, relaxation and health. You can also create thousands of your own personal affirmations for any areas of your life.

Some software programs flash these messages, which include audio, on your computer screen for just milliseconds to reach the subliminal level of the mind. You may want to give them a try.

Are you comfortable physically?

In order to keep stress at bay, dress as comfortably as you can within your employer's dress code. I'm not advocating going to work in jeans and a baggie t-shirt if your employer bans this type of clothing. But don't constrict yourself unnecessarily. If you're a woman and have to wear dress shoes, you may want to choose flat ones instead of heels.

Beyond that, make sure your chair is comfortable and that the temperature is within a certain comfortable range. Don't wait until your environment becomes intolerable to make changes. Being physically comfortable reduces your stress more than you can imagine.

Acknowledge your limits

Don't worry about appearing weak or something less than a superstar. Recognize what you can do and what you can't. Some individuals waste their time in a vain attempt to control events or – even worse — other people in order to accomplish their goals. This never works.

Steven Covey said it best in his *7 Habits of Highly Effective People* when he told us to know what we can change and what we can't. Then focus on those items we have control over.

When a stressful situation is put in front of you, ask yourself this question first: "Is this really my problem?" If you answer no, then walk away from it.

If you discover it's yours to tackle, then tackle first things first. Identify any steps you can take immediately to remedy it. And once you have handled it to your satisfaction, set it aside and be confident in your actions. Don't try to second guess yourself.

Don't be afraid to compromise

You can avoid unwanted stress by learning how to compromise. Many individuals get upset and stressed out when someone acts other they believe they should. Some get upset when their ideas aren't adopted in whole. *Compromise.* It's much less stressful than confrontation, and it goes a long way in reducing your stress.

These are steps you can take this very moment in your daily affairs. Here are some other activities you can begin today — or in the near future.

Ever tried yoga?

For the longest time, this stress-busting practice wasn't recognized in the Western world despite its illustrious history in the East. In fact, yoga is a practice that dates back at least 5,000 years. It is, without a doubt, the oldest form of self-development.

Only recently have people in other parts of the world embraced this activity. Some employers actually offer yoga to their employees. This trend is especially popular in Great Britain. These employers know that workers who aren't stressed out are not only healthier, but more productive and more creative. Instead of dealing with their stress, these employees are busy dealing with the details of their jobs.

Many of the techniques used today — separate from this ancient practice — are actually derived originally from yoga. They include controlled breathing and meditation, mental imagery, and stretching and physical movement.

Interestingly, the word yoga comes from the same root as the word *yoke*. And this isn't just a coincidence. Yoke means to bring together. Yoga, in a very real way, does just that. It brings together the mind, body and spirit.

Many individuals use yoga as a method of transformation, but more than that, its popularity can be attributed to its effectiveness in stress management and improving your physical health.

What exactly can yoga do?

You'd be surprised at the far-reaching stress-reduction effects and physiological benefits this gentle activity brings. A few of yoga's advantages include:

- Reduction of stress

- Improved sleeping habits

- Reduction of cortisol levels

- Allergy symptom relief

- Asthma symptom relief

- Decrease in blood pressure

- Slower heart rate

- Reduction in anxiety

- Reduction in muscle tension

- Increased strength

- Improved flexibility

- Slowing of the aging process

Before you even begin to think that part of yoga is contorting yourself like a pretzel, let me set you straight. There are a large variety of poses, many of which aren't of the pretzel-bending sort. And this is especially true as a beginner. The moves are simple yet highly effect at relieving stress.

Basically, yoga is the stretching of the body into a variety of poses. At the same time, you breathe slowly and in a controlled manner. Ironically, your body not only realizes a natural state of relaxation, but it's also energized at the same time.

But the results aren't just all in your head. Recent research confirms that your physical body also undergoes a transformation. As you practice yoga, your body releases high levels of a chemical called serotonin, a substance that induces feelings of well-being.

When you start looking into yoga classes, you'll discover that there are many different types of yoga. Some practices have goals that target spiritual transformation; others simply aim to help you stretch, relax and reduce stress. When you seek a class, be sure to ask what type of yoga the class involves and its ultimate aim.

If you're searching specifically for a style that reduces your stress without any spiritual implications, a Hatha yoga class would be a good one to try.

Besides attending classes, there are many DVDs and books available that will show you the various poses as well. Look for a beginner yoga DVD.

Meditation

Another form of relaxation is meditation. Not surprisingly, meditation is rooted in the practice of yoga. But, you don't need to learn yoga to meditate. Meditation, many people are finding, is a powerful relaxation tool. Not only that, this simple practice can bring about positive health changes in your body.

Thankfully, you don't need to be a Yogi to mediate. A Yogi is a member of such eastern religions as Buddhism, Hinduism, and Taoism who practices the ancient art of meditation.

No, to reap the real benefits of mediation, you don't need to subscribe to any religion or even have any desire to seek a spiritual plateau.

It's true that thousands of years ago, meditation was once confined to the realms of the spiritual elite. Typically, the word meditation conjures up an image of a Buddhist monk in a cave contemplating the meaning of life. One of the best known of these monks is Milarepa, who spent years isolated in a cave in the mountains of Tibet seeking enlightenment.

Enlightenment? Though running off to a cave may sound appealing when you're overwhelmed and barraged with a myriad of stresses, it's rather impractical. Besides, when you return from that cold, damp cave, the pressures you left behind are probably still going to exist.

Meditation: simple and inexpensive

Meditation — once you become accustomed to it — is simple to perform and inexpensive. It doesn't require any special equipment, although some individuals invest in soothing music to help them slip into a meditative state.

If you're still hesitant because you think you'll have to contort your legs pretzel-like into the classic, but uncomfortable-looking full lotus position, don't worry. You don't.

You can meditate anywhere in any position. There are walking meditations. In fact there's a practice of this art that you perform while you walk through a large labyrinth. You can meditate while you're riding for the bus or the subway, in the doctor's waiting room, or even in the midst of a business meeting.

Is meditation some hocus-pocus trick?

Many people still have the mistaken idea that clearing your mind and relaxing—which is all this is—is some hocus-pocus magic trick. It isn't. More and more it's becoming an acknowledged mind-body complementary medicine, recognized even by allopathic physicians.

Complementary medicine is any useful aid you perform *in addition* to conventional medicine. For you, as a sufferer of leaky gut syndrome, it doesn't mean you abandon your elimination diet or your other treatments. It merely means that you meditate along with every other therapy.

This form of stress-reduction works because it takes your physical body into a heightened state of relaxation and it calms your mind. Your goal is to eliminate that jumbled stream of thoughts that are racing through your brain. When you can reach this state you'll be utterly impressed with just how good you feel.

The best aspect of meditation is that the marvelous relaxing effect doesn't end when you've completed your meditation session. A simple session — which lasts a minimum of 15 or 20 minutes — can help you tackle the rest of the day no matter what's thrown at you.

Mayoclinic.com refers to the effects of meditation as "clearing away the information overload that builds up every day and contributes to your stress." I couldn't have said it better. How often are you preoccupied with what happened in the past or the "what ifs" of the future. Meditation puts you squarely in the present — where all is calm.

The emotional benefits of this ancient practice include:

- Viewing your stressful situations differently

- Creating a clear stress-management program

- Increasing an awareness of yourself

- Learning to focus on the present moment

- Decreasing negative emotions

That's really only a small — but vital — part of the power of meditation.

Modern research is also revealing that this practice can actually improve certain medical disorders. In addition to helping you conquer leaky gut syndrome, it has been known to help a wide array of health problems including:

- Allergies

- Drug abuse

- Alcohol abuse

- Anxiety

- Sleep issues

- Asthma

- Pain

- Binge eating

- High blood pressure

- Cancer

- Heart disease

- Depression

- Fatigue

Believe it or not, researchers at Harvard University estimate that stress accounts for fifty to ninety percent of all doctor's visits.

The following statistics are really quite eye-opening. Stress is cited for nearly twenty percent of all the absenteeism in the workplace. It's the cause of nearly forty percent of companies' turnover rate in employees.

Not only that, but it's also responsible for approximately sixty percent of all workplace accidents and nearly thirty percent of both short- and long-term disabilities.

No, you're not alone if you're feeling the modern-day pressures of stress.

How meditation helps

It may seem like it's too easy. Sit quietly, calm your mind, and help to heal your body. But it really can be that easy. Research is uncovering some surprising results.

Let's talk about high blood pressure first. It's one of the first health conditions that modern research realized can be helped through meditative practices. It's especially useful to people who have moderately high blood pressure. This finding has been proven over and over again during the last quarter century. For some people, their systolic readings —the top number — are actually reduced by 25 mmHg or more.

In another clinical study, those individuals with chronic pain exhibited a reduction of nearly fifty percent in their symptoms through meditation. That's an amazing result, but the following finding is even more remarkable. This reduction lasted for some up to four years following the initial meditation training.

There are thousands of other studies on the medical benefits of meditation—far too many to cite here. But you get the idea.

Choose your form of meditation

What? There are different types of meditation? Exactly. That's one of the beauties of this practice. It meets your needs wherever you may be — and whatever level you're on.

One of the most popular ways to meditate is through a technique called guided meditation, or guided imagery or visualization. With this form, you create mental images of places or specific situations that you find relaxing.

To be most effective, use as many senses as possible. Imagine not only the visual setting, filling in as many details as you can, but try to smell the sea air if you're imagining a beach. Recreate the sounds of your scene — birds singing, waves lapping. Even try to feel the textures of your location — the sand between your toes, the feel of walking barefoot.

Many people find a class and are led by a guide or a specific teacher when they use this technique. And that may be how you want to start. Or you may want to buy a CD that guides you, such as The Soul of Healing Meditations by Deepak Chopra. Or a book such as Healing and Transformation through Self-Guided Imagery by Leslie Davenport

Grab a mantra and meditate

Others meditate with the aid of what's called a *mantra*. Here, you silently repeat a calming word or phrase to help you focus. The word can be as simple as love or peace. Or if you're more spiritual, you may want to repeat a word or phrase you find as part of your religious practice. Many use "shalom."

Then there's mindfulness meditation, which is based on… well, being mindful. It's really all about increasing your awareness and your acceptance of living in the moment.

In this form, you focus your attention on what you experience during your meditation session. You notice the rhythm of your breathing, for example. Or instead of clearing your mind of thoughts, observe the thoughts and emotions. Then allow them to pass with passing judgment on them.

There are still two more forms of meditation, both of these incorporating physical movements. The first is Qi gong. In addition to meditation and physical movement, it also involves performing breathing exercises.

You're probably wondering exactly why it's called this. Qi gong is an ancient Chinese healing and energy tradition. The aim of these exercises — both the physical and the breathing — is to "cleanse, strengthen, and circulate the life energy." In Chinese, your life energy is called Qi or Chi.

This practice not only leads to better health and vitality, according to proponents, but it also produces a tranquil mindset. Just as with other forms of meditation, research shows that Qi gong can help a wide variety of health problems. These include asthma, fibromyalgia, arthritis, headaches, pain, cancer, chronic fatigue, cardiovascular disease, and even cancer.

Step into meditation

You can start a simple mediation practice right now. You just need to follow these very simple steps. Of course, if you decide to progress farther into this practice, you may want to take a class in order to meditate with others.

Or you may decide to buy a beginner book on the topic to learn more about it. I like *Meditation for Dummies* because it starts at the very beginning level and comes in both the book and CD versions. I'm not crazy about the "Dummies" labels for all their books; I think it's a putdown (but, obviously it must be working as a marketing tool), and I have to say the books are great.

Location. Location. Location.

It can't be said enough. You need to seek out a quiet place. This means no television in the background and preferably no radio as well. If you want music, use something that is recommended for this practice. It will relax you without interrupting you.

Good posture

There aren't many rules in this practice, but just about all practitioners agree: mediate with a straight back. Some individuals lie down during their meditation. You may try this if you like. But be aware that you're much more likely to fall asleep when you're in that position than to actually have a meditative session — especially when you're just beginning.

Center yourself

It's difficult to meditate right after work when your mind is still racing. Quiet yourself first. Give yourself time to unwind from anything in your day that is pressing on your mind. You'll find that it's a lot easier to clear your mind.

Or you can meditate first thing in the morning as a way to start your day. Oprah, for example, says she meditates for forty-five minutes before she begins her busy day.

Breathing is the key

Believe it or not, how we breathe affects our mind. One of the tricks to effective meditation is to concentrate on your breathing.

This, in a nutshell, is the most powerful aspect of meditation. You need to be fully conscious of your breathing. Many individuals imagine they're breathing in peace as they inhale.

As you concentrate on your breathing, try to set all other thoughts aside. If a problem crops up in your thinking, gently whisk it away. Continue to concentrate on your breath.

Calming the mind: it won't happen overnight

This last step is the most difficult. Here's a big hint: calming your mind completely will not happen on your first attempt. You may find yourself busy clearing thoughts that creep into your mind. This is normal. Don't react or get upset. Just keep gently pushing them away. Eventually, with enough sessions, clearing your mind will become easier.

And don't worry that, just because you can't clear your mind completely in the beginning, you're not receiving any healing benefits. You are.

You're well on your way to learning the ancient healing art of meditation. You'll be amazed how quickly this can change your perspective. You'll also be pleased as you notice the stresses of the day are less apt to zap your energy.

Guaranteed stress-buster: exercise

I know I'm promoting a sometimes unpopular activity. Many individuals try hard to avoid exercise at all costs. In some ways, that's understandable. After you come home from work, mentally and physically drained, you really just want to sit down and kick your feet up.

We all feel like that. But our first instincts — and deepest desire — in this instance isn't necessarily what's best for us. In reality, we'd all feel much better if we would do some physical activity.

At the very least, performing physical activity helps to relieve the stress that normally burdens you by the end of the day.

Exercise not only de-stresses you, but it improves your health. What you might not have realized, though, is that better health can help you get through your day. It's nothing but a win-win situation.

Need a little prodding to get off that sofa? Let's start with the word *endorphins*. Exercise boosts the production of endorphins. These are neurotransmitters in your brain, which in the simplest terms, just make you feel good.

You've heard the term *runner's high?* It's really the feeling a person gets when more endorphins are in your system. But the beauty of this is that you don't need to run to experience it. Any prolonged physical activity will give you the same feeling.

The corollary to the improved production of endorphins also improves your mood. Depressed? Take some time to exercise—even something as simple as a walk. You don't even have to take a vigorous walk to experience a better mood. The next time you come home from work give it a try. You may be surprised at the result.

Do you have trouble sleeping at night, tossing and turning? Does your mind refuse to shut off, running through the day's events and even tomorrow's? Try some exercise and you'll see that those sleepless nights are a thing of the past.

And when you sleep better, you'll discover you feel less stress. And it can give you a renewed command over your body — and your life.

Getting started: it's easier than you think

As always, before you start any exercise program — even a simple walking regimen — consult your doctor. This is especially true if you have diabetes. O2nce you get the green light from your physician, then you can begin your new life.

Don't start out at full speed. You may be tempted to jump into an exercise program quickly and thoroughly. It's best, though, to start slowly. Even physical activity at a low level is better than none. And you'll feel better even with only a little movement if your body isn't accustomed to it – guaranteed.

Your goal is thirty minutes a day. If you're out of shape, you may have trouble doing even this much. Don't despair; build up to this. With just a little determination and discipline, you'll be able to work your way up to a half hour.

Choose an activity you like. Exercise is exercise. Your body treats a rousing game of tennis the same as is does a good walk or run. So don't think you're stuck performing some activity that doesn't suit your lifestyle and your preferences. Even time spent in the garden lovingly tending to your plants can be exercise enough to de-stress you.

Once you start your program, make it a habit. This means you make an appointment with yourself and you don't break it. If your employer said he wanted to meet with you Monday at 3 p.m., you wouldn't ignore him, would you? Then don't blow off your daily appointment with exercise.

Now that's easier said than done, you say. Perhaps at the beginning you may think that. But, once you get started, you'll want that feel-good-all-over effect that physical activity brings. Eventually (and this may be difficult to believe), your body will tell you it *needs* the activity.

If you have trouble starting and sustaining a program, consider enlisting the help of a good friend. Set aside time for the two of you to walk with each other. It might be easier to keep your appointment if you know somebody is sitting on a park bench waiting for you.

And you may just discover that when you exercise with a friend, you're more motivated and more committed.

Some individuals start with one form of activity only to find they tire of it. If this should happen to you, don't give up. Perhaps what you need to do is find a second form of exercise. And then you can alternate between say walking and swimming during the week. Give it some thought if you think you're getting bored.

Okay. Now you're ready to start your de-stressing program through physical activity. Go ahead; give it a try. You'll discover a whole new wonderful relaxing world ahead of you.

And the beauty of it all, you'll notice that the symptoms associated with your leaky gut syndrome are dramatically reduced.

Conclusion

You and I are coming to the end of our journey. You've learned, as I did, that Leaky Gut Syndrome is nothing less than an invisible thief—a stealth disorder masquerading as any number of other disorders—robbing you of your health and energy.

You've also learned that diagnosing this disorder can be quite complicated because of the sneakiness of this syndrome.

If you suffer from leaky gut, I hope you can now see light at the end of the tunnel. A solution is waiting for you.

Treat leaky gut syndrome naturally

You now have tools at your disposal and resources at your command to cure leaky gut syndrome naturally, without the need for harsh prescription drugs.

While this book provides you with the necessary tools to embark on a healing program, you've really only just begun your journey.

If you start with these suggestions and continue working at it, you CAN take back what leaky gut stole from you—your health and happiness. You deserve it!

"The greatest wealth is health."
Virgil

Appendix
A Sample Leaky Gut Syndrome Elimination Diet

The following is a sample elimination diet. Here you'll find some guidelines as to what to eliminate in order to ease the symptoms of leaky gut syndrome.

You don't necessarily need to follow it word for word. You can easily choose the foods that give you the most trouble on the list and start with that. Any steps you take toward eating healthier are an excellent start.

The following is a list of foods that you should stop eating for one month to allow your body to begin to heal. These foods are commonly the most troublesome for many people with leaky gut syndrome

- Bananas

- Beans

- Bread

- Caffeine

- Chocolate

- Citrus fruits

- Corn

- Dairy products

- Eggs

- Flour

- Gluten grains (wheat, spelt, kamut, rye, and barley)

- Honey

- Kiwi

- Millet

- Mushroom

- Nightshade vegetables (eggplant, peppers, tomatoes)

- Oats

- Papaya

- Peanuts

- Pineapple

- Soy products

- Strawberries

- Vanilla extract

- Vinegar

- Yeast

Here is a list of foods that you may eat. Choose the foods you enjoy most so the diet doesn't get to be monotonous or too restrictive for your tastes. It's possible, believe it or not, to perform an elimination diet and not really miss the foods you can't eat at all.

Stay with this list for a month. Your body will begin to adjust and then you can begin — slowly — to add foods to one at a time to your diet.

- Amaranth

- Apples

- Apricots

- Avocados

- Beets

- Berries (except strawberries)

- Bok choy

- Brussels Sprouts

- Carrots

- Cherries

- Cilantro

- Coconut milk
- Dandelion Greens
- Figs
- Grapes
- Kale
- Lettuce
- Nectarines
- Olive oil
- Onions
- Parsnips
- Peaches
- Pears
- Pine nuts
- Plums
- Pumpkin seeds
- Quinoa
- Rice, brown and wild
- Spinach
- Sprouts
- Sunflower seeds

Phase 2 of a Sample Elimination Diet

Add the following foods to the allowable list. Add one food at a time. Wait three days before you add another one. If the food gives you an allergic reaction or your body doesn't react well to it, stay away from it for another month.

- Bananas

- Beans

- Chicken

- Fish

- Nightshade vegetables

- Papaya

- Pineapple

- Soy

- Turkey

Phase 3 of a Sample Elimination Diet

Add the following foods, again, one at a time in three-day increments. If you get an adverse reaction, then eliminate the food for another month.

- Alcohol

- Caffeine

- Chocolate

- Kiwi

- Oranges

- Peanuts

- Sesame seeds

- Strawberries

- Sugar, refined

- Pea

Phase 4 of a Sample Elimination Diet

Add the following foods, again, one at a time in three-day increments. If you get an adverse reaction, then eliminate it for another month.

- Bread

- Corn

- Eggs

- Millet

- Yeast

- Gluten grains

- Dairy products

References & Resources

Books

Leaky Gut Cure
Karen Brimeyer

Total Renewal: 7 Key Steps to Resilience, Vitality, and Long-Term Health
Frank Lipman and Stephanie Gunning

Leaky Gut Syndrome
Elizabeth Lipski

Your Plan for a Balanced Life
James M. Rippe, M.D. and Thomas Nelson

The Detox Strategy: Vibrant Health in 5 Easy Steps
Brenda Watson with Leonard Smith, M.D.

Healing and Transformation through Self-Guided Imagery
Leslie Davenport

Books

Meditation for Dummies
Stephan Bodian

Yoga for Dummies
Georg Feuerstein

Yoga for Every Body
Paul Harvey

CDs and DVDs

Music for Zen Meditation and Other Joys

The Unexplainable Store
(Meditation, Affirmations, Abundance)

The Soul of Healing Meditations
Deepak Chopra

Yoga for Beginners
Barbara Benagh

Software

Mind Zoom
(Incredible affirmations and abundance technology!)

Websites

Leaky Gut Syndrome,
http://www.drkaslow.com/html/leaky_gut.html,
accessed 21 Mar 11.

Adrenal Fatigue/Adrenal Exhaustion,
http://thyroid.about.com/cs/endocrinology/a/adrenal
fatigue.htm,
accessed 25 Mar 11.

Non-Steroidal Anti-Inflammatory Drugs,
http://en.wikipedia.org/wiki/Non-steroidal_anti-
inflammatory_drug,
accessed 26 Mar 11.

The Human Digestive System,
http://www.constipationopia.com/the-human-
digestive-system.html,
accessed 27 Mar 11.

Anaphylaxis,
http://www.ncbi.nlm.nih.gov/pubmedhealth/PMH000
1847/accessed 27 Mar 11.

Cholecystokinin,
http://www.mayoclinic.com/health/drug-information/DR600365,
accessed 28 Mar 11.

Parasites,
http://www.cdc.gov/parasites/,
accessed 28 Mar 11.

Butyric Acid: an Ancient Controller of Metabolism, Inflammation and Stress Resistance,
http://wholehealthsource.blogspot.com/2009/12/butyric-acid-ancient-controller-of.html,
accessed 28 Mar 11.

Testing for Leaky Gut Syndrome,
http://www.leakygut.co.uk/testing.htm,
accessed 29 Mar 11.

Healing a leaky gut naturally,
http://www.stopleakygut.com/healing,
accessed 29 Mar 11.

Leaky gut syndrome treatment,
http://www.ei-resource.org/treatment-options/treatment-information/leaky-gut-syndrome-treatment/,
accessed 29 Mar 11.

Digestion and GI Health,
http://www.womentowomen.com/digestionandgihealt
h/leakygutsyndrome-
intestinalpermeability.aspx#healingleakygut,
accessed 29 Mar 11.

Gut Dysbiosis,
http://www.regenerativenutrition.com/natural-
supplements-cure-gut-dysbiosis.asp,
accessed 29 Mar 11.

Healing with probiotics,
http://www.healingdaily.com/detoxification-
diet/probiotics.htm,
accessed 1 Apr 11.

How to Use a Rotation Diet,
http://www.food-allergy.org/rotation.html,
accessed 2 Apr 11.

FOS—Fructooligosaccharides,
http://www.naturaltherapypages.com.au/article/FOS_
Fructooligosaccharides,
accessed 2 April 11.

Leaky Gut Syndrome Treatment,
http://www.ei-resource.org/treatment-options/treatment-information/leaky-gut-syndrome-treatment/,
accessed 3 April 11.

Straight from the Leaky Gut,
http://www.hfldirect.com/index.php?main_page=index&cPath=124_188_192,
accessed 3 Apr 11

Index

A

B

C

D

E

F

G

H

I

Q

Qi gong, 101
quality of life, 13
quick starter's guide, 47

R

radiation treatment, 30
relaxation, 90, 94, 95, 97
root, 75, 78, 93
ROS, 56
rotation diet, 43, 48, 54

S

Secretory IgA, 22, 28
sensitivity, 35
serotonin, 94
sleep issues, 98
sleep problems, 41, 85
slippery elm, 72, 73
software, 90, 91
steroids, 30, 49
stress, 20, 31, 40, 57, 67, 79, 80, 81, 82, 83, 84, 85, 86, 87, 88, 89, 90, 91, 92, 93, 94, 95, 97, 98, 99, 104, 105, 106
sugar, 50, 51, 53, 55, 59
sun, 31, 57
symptoms, 11, 12, 13, 16, 17, 18, 20, 29, 30, 34, 37, 41, 51, 52, 54, 55, 59, 70, 72, 83, 85, 99, 107, 113

T

tea, 53, 73, 74, 75, 78
tincture, 76, 78, 79
tissue toxicity, 18
Total Body Cleanse, 68
toxins, 16, 17, 18, 19, 22, 25, 28, 43, 49, 59, 67, 68
treatment, 14, 25, 44, 53, 74, 77, 78, 126, 128

U

ulcerative colitis, 24, 38
ulcers, 24, 72, 73

V

Y

Z

More Books by Regency Publications

No More MOO: The Dairy-Free and Lactose-Free Guide to Living Well with Lactose Intolerance

Savannah Paris

Write eBooks: Make Money: The No-Fear Guide to Writing Your Own Money-Spinning eBook

April Manning

Find them now on Amazon.

More about...

No More Moo: The Dairy-Free and Lactose-Free Guide to Living Well with Lactose Intolerance

Many people with leaky gut also suffer from lactose intolerance. Often the two go hand in hand. **No More Moo** delivers straight talk on the causes and effects of lactose intolerance and how to heal it.

If you suffer from lactose intolerance, or you just want to avoid dairy products for a healthier diet, this book is for you. Millions of Americans are lactose intolerant—some with severe, painful symptoms—but it doesn't have to be this way

Learn more about lactose intolerance as you strive for ultimate health and wellness. **No More Moo** may be for you.

[Excerpt]
No More MOO:
The Dairy-Free and Lactose-Free Guide to Living Well with Lactose Intolerance

Savannah Paris

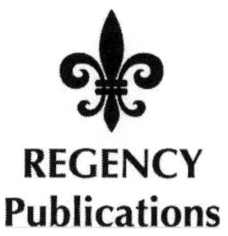

REGENCY
Publications

Introduction
My Story

All I had to do was drive thirteen miles to get home—but I didn't make it.

The evening had begun innocently enough. As president of a professional writer's association, I was the host of our annual awards ceremony. As master of ceremonies, my job was to keep the audience entertained, move the show along and hand out awards to happy winners.

The event was held at an exclusive, upscale restaurant, which provided an appealing selection of appetizers and hors d'oeuvres. People hovered around the tables, talking, eating, drinking and socializing.

Because I had to prepare for my hosting duties, I quickly choose two appetizers that looked appealing and took a few small bites. I worked for about a half hour behind the scenes. Just as I took my place on stage, I was stunned by a wave of stomach cramping that took my breath away.

The only thing I could think of was to get to a restroom, but then the spotlight was, literally, on me. Thankfully adrenaline kicked in and I began the show, which lasted for more than an hour. As soon as the show was over, my pumped-up adrenaline vanished and the painful cramping came back stronger than ever.

I found a restroom in time and, after an attack of diarrhea, the pain stopped. But unfortunately, as I started driving home, my stomach cramping returned with a vengeance. Because I had just driven onto a long causeway (a raised highway over a bay with water on both sides) there were no exits, no stops and no chance of finding a restroom.

The cramping got so bad I had difficulty pushing the gas pedal down; I felt nauseated and rapidly broke out into a cold sweat from the pain. My only goal was to get to a restroom as soon as possible. When I was finally able to exit the causeway, I spotted a restaurant and quickly pulled into the parking lot. This is extremely embarrassing to admit, but I didn't make it to the restroom in time.

That was my life with lactose intolerance. Apparently the small amount of hidden dairy in those few bites was enough to do me in that day.

I've written this book because I don't want this to be your life, too. I don't want you to suffer the discomfort and sometimes humiliation of this distressing and often painful condition because *you don't have to*. Wherever you are on the lactose intolerance spectrum—from mild to severe, you can learn to live a symptom-free life and enjoy a lactose-free lifestyle.

Inside this book, you'll find the information and techniques I used to rid myself of the symptoms of lactose intolerance. Whether you suffer a little or a lot from lactose intolerance, **No More MOO** is written for you.

Chapter One
Lactose Intolerance 101

Got milk?

There's no shortage of milk in the United States and there's no shortage of people who love it. For many of us, it's unthinkable to have our coffee or morning cereal without milk. Yes, we love our milk—although, unfortunately, sometimes it doesn't love us.

If you suffer from mild lactose intolerance, milk and dairy products can produce unpleasant symptoms. If you suffer from severe lactose intolerance, like I did, milk and dairy are more than a little bothersome—they're the enemy—and they take no prisoners.

Lactose defined

What is lactose? Some people incorrectly believe that lactose is a form of fat that's found in dairy products and milk. Lactose is actually a sugar—not a fat. It's often referred to as a "natural sugar" because it's found specifically in milk that's produced by mammals.

If you eat dairy products, you're consuming lactose.

And you may not know this, but if you're eating and drinking alternative milk and dairy products, you're also consuming lactose. Any milk produced by a mammal will cause symptoms; so substituting other types of milk— such as goat's milk or sheep's milk—unfortunately, isn't the solution. Yogurt made from sheep's milk, for example, actually contains more lactose than cow's milk.

Important: lactose intolerance is **NOT** a milk allergy

Lactose intolerance is your intestine's reaction to milk **sugar**. A milk allergy is a systemic immune reaction against milk **proteins**.

Some symptoms of milk allergy can be similar to lactose intolerance symptoms. If you have any symptoms, you could be lactose intolerance, have a milk allergy, or both.

Lactose intolerance plain and simple

First, here's some basic information:

Lactose intolerance—also known as "lactose malabsorption" or "lactase deficiency"—is a condition where the body is unable to digest lactose (milk sugar).

Lactose has two main components: *glucose* (the type of sugar your body can easily digest) and *galactose*. When you consume dairy products, your body is faced with the job of splitting lactose into these two components.

Got lactase?

Lactase, which is manufactured in the lining of the small intestine, is the only enzyme in your digestive system that can break down **lactose**.

Ideally, you should have enough **lactase** to continually and regularly break down and absorb **lactose**. But, if you're suffering from lactose intolerance this, regrettably, isn't the case.

What causes it?

There are three main types of lactose intolerance:

Primary lactose intolerance:

This is the most common form of the condition. The lactase gene expression turns off in childhood and, over time, your body can stop producing adequate amounts of this essential enzyme. It may take years for symptoms to appear, which occur usually in adulthood.

Secondary lactose intolerance:

If you become ill from a disease that affects your small intestine—like inflammatory conditions, bacterial, viral or parasitic infections—you can become lactose intolerant. Fortunately, in most cases, this lactose intolerance disappears in a few weeks.

Congenital lactase deficiency:

This is a rare case in which a baby is born without the ability to produce lactase. Infants born with this condition will remain lactose intolerant throughout their lives.

Note: Some *premature* infants are born lactose intolerant. But, this type of lactose intolerance is generally temporary. Once the baby's GI tract is more mature, he or she will begin producing a normal amount of lactase. At that point, the baby will be able to drink milk and other lactose products with no problems.

What happens when you don't have enough lactase?

How much dairy you can eat depends on how much lactase enzyme your body makes. If you have little or no lactase, your body labors when you eat lactose. The less lactase your body produces, the more severe your symptoms will be. If lactase isn't available in any form, your body will no longer be able to digest and absorb lactose.

So what happens when your body can't digest lactose? In short, when your body doesn't have enough lactase to thoroughly break down lactose in your small intestine, it reaches the large intestine intact. When this undigested material enters the large intestine, it serves as food for bacteria dwelling there. As the bacteria feed upon the undigested milk sugar, gases and irritating acids are produced creating unpleasant and sometime severe symptoms.

What are the symptoms? They're pretty much hard to ignore:

Bloating

Intestinal cramping

Acute abdominal pain

A stomach that gurgles

Gas

Diarrhea

Vomiting

The bloating occurs due to increased gas production in the digestive tract. Yuck. And the other symptoms follow.

How do I know if what I have is lactose intolerance?

This is important:

There may be other reasons why you could be experiencing all or some of these symptoms. There can be a number of *other* conditions you may be suffering from that aren't remotely related to lactose intolerance. That's why it's essential to know their cause. Don't guess; you need to be one hundred percent sure of what's actually affecting your health.

Chapter Two
Diagnosing Lactose Intolerance

You may be able to diagnose lactose intolerance yourself. The simplest test is called the "Milk Challenge" test.

The milk challenge

The milk challenge is an easy way of diagnosing lactose intolerance. To take the test, you fast overnight, and then drink a glass of milk in the morning. After that, you have nothing to eat or drink for three to five hours. If you're lactose intolerant, the milk should produce symptoms within several hours of ingestion.

But this test may not be conclusive. If you're not sure, you can choose to try the next test—Dairy Elimination.

Dairy Elimination test

Try eliminating all sources of dairy products and other products that may contain lactose for one to two weeks. Believe me; I understand this is no ordinary undertaking.

To test myself, I eliminated all dairy and processed foods, ate only vegetables and meat, and drank soy milk for two weeks. (I knew for sure these items didn't contain lactose.) My symptoms went away.

To reintroduce dairy, I ate a big bowl of my favorite chocolate ice cream. I didn't know it at the time, but many ice cream manufacturers add additional lactose to ice cream to make it creamier. Wow, it didn't take long. My lactose intolerance symptoms came back in less than an hour. I decided I didn't need to pursue any further testing. Without a doubt, I was sure I was lactose intolerant.

If this one- to two-week regimen of just meat, vegetables and a milk alternative (such as soy or almond milk) is too difficult for you, you can try a less restricted diet. But, if you decide to go for this self-test, it will take some detective work on your part to eliminate all dairy products. Dairy is often hidden in hundreds of food products and medications. (We'll discuss how to spot hidden lactose in Chapter Three.)

After one to two weeks on this less-restricted diet, if your symptoms disappear, you're most likely lactose intolerant. But, even if you're symptoms DON'T go away, you STILL may be lactose intolerant. If you accidently consumed lactose—even though you were trying hard to avoid it—your self-test will be inconclusive.

If your particular case is hard to diagnose, consider seeing a doctor. He or she can prescribe medical tests to determine lactose intolerance.

Before you take these tests, your doctor probably will ask you to take the one- to two-week Dairy Elimination test first. So, if you've avoided it up until this point, it's better to get it over with. Then, he or she will use one or more conclusive tests to confirm the diagnosis.

There are two main tests:

Hydrogen Breath test

The hydrogen breath test is the preferred and most common method. It measures the amount of hydrogen in the air you breathe out. The test is pretty simple and noninvasive. This test is done at an outpatient clinic or doctor's office. Before the test, you'll be asked to do a selective fast. (Your doctor will tell you what not to eat or drink before the test.)

When the testing begins, you'll be instructed to breathe into a balloon-type container. Next, you'll be asked to drink a flavored liquid containing lactose. Then, over a period of hours, samples of your breathe will be collected again and your hydrogen levels will be measured. Normally very little hydrogen should be present in your system so, if the test results show you have low levels of hydrogen, you DON'T have lactose intolerance.

But if your body has trouble breaking down and absorbing lactose, your breath hydrogen levels will increase. If your hydrogen levels are high, it's likely you have lactose intolerance. If your doctor isn't satisfied with the results, he or she might order more tests.

Note: The hydrogen breath test is generally reserved for older children and adults. It's not performed on infants because the testing technique (the use of a lactose-filled fluid and selective fasting) can lead to diarrhea in infants.

Lactose tolerance blood test

The lactose tolerance blood test looks for glucose in your blood because your body creates glucose when lactose breaks down.

For this test, you won't be allowed to eat or drink anything after midnight. After your overnight fast, you'll get a lactose-filled liquid to drink. Then blood samples are taken over two hours to measure your blood sugar levels.

After you drink the lactose solution, if you don't have lactose intolerance, you'll be able to digest the lactose drink and your blood sugar level will increase considerably. But, if you're lactose intolerant, your blood sugar level will stay the same.

How to test for a milk allergy

As mentioned, lactose intolerance is often confused with a milk allergy. Here's a way to test for it...

End of Sample

5744950R00084

Printed in Great Britain
by Amazon.co.uk, Ltd.,
Marston Gate.